Healing Together

Healing Together

MOTIVATIONAL INTERVIEWING FOR HEALTHCARE PROVIDERS

Carol Berger and Lynette Dixon

cognella
SAN DIEGO

Bassim Hamadeh, CEO and Publisher
Amanda Martin, Executive Publisher
Alverne Ball, Project Editor
Rachel Kahn, Production Editor
Jess Estrella, Senior Graphic Designer
Laura Duncan, Licensing Specialist
Tiffany Mok, Senior Content Marketing Specialist
Natalie Piccotti, Director of Marketing
Kassie Graves, Senior Vice President, Editorial
Alia Bales, Director of Project Editorial & Production

Printed in the United States of America.

BRIEF CONTENTS

DETAILED CONTENTS

INTRODUCTION

According to Gallup's annual "**Most Honest and Ethical Professional Poll,**" nurses have ranked number one for 22 years and counting with 78% of respondents rating nurses as "high" or "very high" when it comes to honesty or ethical standards, and medical doctors come in at fifth place with 56%. Looking at the results, veterinarians, engineers, and dentists were thought to be more ethical and honest than medical doctors in the 2023 poll (Gallup, 2024).

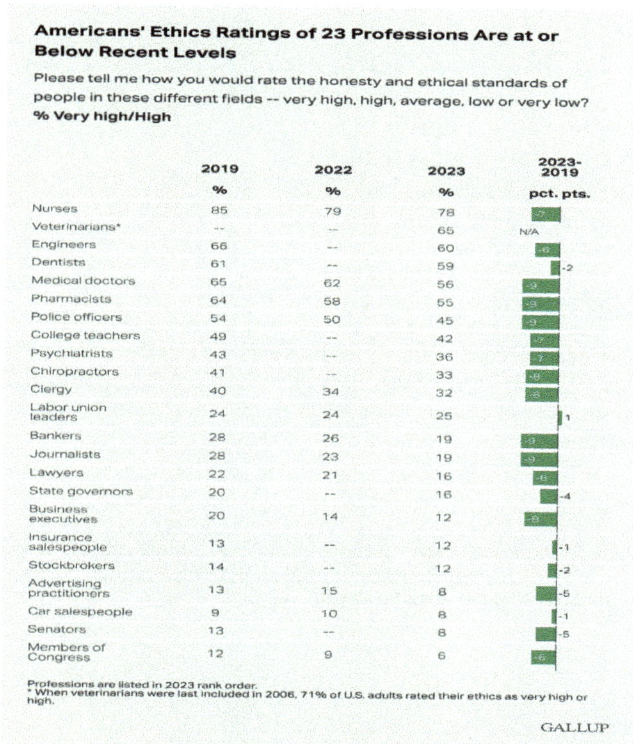

Americans' Ethics Ratings of 23 Professions Are at or Below Recent Levels

Please tell me how you would rate the honesty and ethical standards of people in these different fields -- very high, high, average, low or very low?
% Very high/High

	2019 %	2022 %	2023 %	2023-2019 pct. pts.
Nurses	85	79	78	-7
Veterinarians*	--	--	65	N/A
Engineers	66	--	60	-6
Dentists	61	--	59	-2
Medical doctors	65	62	56	-9
Pharmacists	64	58	55	-9
Police officers	54	50	45	-9
College teachers	49	--	42	-7
Psychiatrists	43	--	36	-7
Chiropractors	41	--	33	-8
Clergy	40	34	32	-8
Labor union leaders	24	24	25	1
Bankers	28	26	19	-9
Journalists	28	23	19	-9
Lawyers	22	21	16	-6
State governors	20	--	16	-4
Business executives	20	14	12	-8
Insurance salespeople	13	--	12	-1
Stockbrokers	14	--	12	-2
Advertising practitioners	13	15	8	-5
Car salespeople	9	10	8	-1
Senators	13	--	8	-5
Members of Congress	12	9	6	-6

Professions are listed in 2023 rank order.
* When veterinarians were last included in 2006, 71% of U.S. adults rated their ethics as very high or high.

GALLUP

Figure I.1 American ethics rating.

To help us understand the mindset of those attracted to the nursing field, we need to look at how the American Nurses Association (2021) defines nursing:

Nursing integrates the art and science of caring and focuses on the protection, promotion, and optimization of health and human functioning, prevention of illness and injury, facilitation of healing and alleviation of suffering through compassionate presence. Nursing is the diagnosis and treatment of human responses and advocacy in the care of individuals, families, groups, communities, and populations in recognition of the connection of all humanity. (p. 1)

It is our hope that, as you read through these chapters, you will gain insight into how to create an environment with your patients that invites healing and engagement. We will show you how to allow your patients to educate *you* about who they are and what they need rather than only having you educate them on changes that you think they need to make. We will also show you multiple techniques that research has shown to be more effective than the "traditional" or "expert" approach. Before we can show you these strategies, we need to open the eyes of your understanding to the patient's experience.

Things to Think About

- What is your patient's story?
- What fears do they bring with them?
- What are your patients' hopes?
- What do they need from you?

References

American Nurses Association. (2021). *Nursing: Scope and standards of practice* (4th ed.).

Gallup. (2024, January 22). *Ethics ratings of nearly all professions down in U.S.* https://news.gallup.com/poll/608903/ethics-ratings-nearly-professions-down.aspx

Figure Credit

Fig. I.1: Gallup, "Americans' Ethics Ratings of 23 Professions Are at or Below Recent Levels," https://news.gallup.com/poll/608903/ethics-ratings-nearly-professions-down.aspx. Copyright © 2024 by Gallup, Inc.

Chapter 1

The Patients' Perspective in Healthcare

Listen to your patient. He is telling you the diagnosis.

—Sir William Osler

In this chapter we want to illustrate the patient's experience as they seek health care in a hospital, while getting test results, or during an exchange with a provider that is less than optimal. We will explore rates of patient satisfaction within the healthcare system, as it is, and we will examine the factors that exist within our current treatment approach that cause them the most frustration. Then we will explore an alternative way of building rapport with a patient that focuses on meeting them where they are with no judgment and utilizing **effective communication techniques** that will empower them and give them ownership in their health care. Furthermore, we will show how research supports this approach as being more effective for patients increasing **patient satisfaction** rates while simultaneously decreasing **provider burnout** by allowing the provider to "fall back in love" with what attracted them to this field in the first place (Shute, 2019).

OBJECTIVES

- Students will gain insight into the patient's experience.
- Students will be able to demonstrate the ability to distinguish between effective and noneffective communication techniques.
- Students will analyze various holistic factors that are involved in the patient experience to include social, cultural, and economic determinants of health.

- Students will be able to recognize and understand how important patient involvement impacts patient engagement.

KEY TERMS AND DEFINITIONS

- **Patient experience:** Includes the emotional, mental, and physical journey a patient undergoes while seeking health care, influenced by the quality of communication and interaction with health care providers.
- **Patient satisfaction:** Patient satisfaction is a measurement of how well health care services meet the expectations, needs, and preferences of the patient.
- **Effective communication techniques:** Effective communication techniques include methods that prioritize listening, empathy, and clarity to empower patients and foster trust.
- **Empathy:** Empathy is the ability to understand and share the feelings of another person, creating a supportive and trusting health care environment.
- **Motivational interviewing:** Motivational interviewing is a collaborative, patient-centered counseling approach that helps patients explore ambivalence to change and find the motivation within themselves to make positive changes in their lives.
- **Sacred space:** A health care setting where patients feel safe, respected, and empowered to be vulnerable and express their concerns to the provider.
- **Health literacy:** Involves a patient's ability to understand, process, and act on health-related information regardless of their literacy status to make informed decisions about their care.
- **Narrative medicine:** An approach that emphasizes listening to a patient's story to understand their experiences to build a deeper connection.
- **Cultural sensitivity and diversity:** A practice of understanding and respecting the cultural, social, and personal backgrounds of patients to provide equitable and inclusive care.
- **Shared decision-making:** A collaborative process whereby health care providers and patients jointly discuss and make decisions about treatment and care plans.
- **Implicit bias in healthcare:** Involves unconscious attitudes or stereotypes that influence a provider's actions and decisions, often leading to disparities in care.
- **Provider burnout:** The emotional and physical exhaustion experienced by providers, often alleviated by adopting patient-centered approaches that reconnect them with their passion for care.

Note to Our Readers

For centuries, in both the fields of nursing and medicine, the term "patient" has been the preferred term to refer to individuals who receive care from a provider. However, in the fields of psychology and counseling, the term "client" is more often the preferred term. This shift began around the 1940s and 50s, with the development of humanistic psychology, popularized by pioneers like Carl Rogers, who is discussed extensively in Chapter 5. The term "client" is preferred for many reasons:

- It indicates a collaborative partnership in which the individual takes an active role rather than simply coming to the provider to passively receive care.
- It is empowering to the client and reinforces the idea that they have autonomy regarding the decision-making process.
- The term "patient" is associated with the medical model, which emphasizes illness and pathology. The term "client" can indicate more of person-centered approach.
- It takes away from the hierarchical relationship that can support power imbalances. Much like a financial advisor who a person comes to for expertise and advice but still retains decision-making power and input over their money, the term "client" creates a relationship in which this type of relationship can take place.

Throughout this book, we have opted to use the word "patient" primarily, although the word "client" appears more frequently both in nursing literature and standardized prelicensure testing (e.g., the NCLEX). You may find some instances when we used the word "client." We want to encourage the provider–patient relationship to be open and collaborative and to contain the principles outlined in this book rather than get hung up on terminology.

The Patient Experience

Carol's Experience

It was another night on the 10th floor of the neurological unit, and I was finishing up my shift. One last med pass, charting and then home—hopefully I would make it home to be able to give the kids baths, read stories, and put them to bed. It had been a long time since I had been done on time; there was always something that came up. One thing I was grateful for was my 12-hour shift would fly by, as there was never enough time to get everything done. But as I entered my next-to-last patient's room, I could see she was crying. I had come to restart her IV, so I thought she was upset, but as she talked, I realized she was scared. I could have ignored her tears and started the IV, hung up the bag of antibiotics, and patted her hand, sticking to my plan to get done on time, but I could not let myself do that. Here was a woman who was frightened of something, and this was why I was here.

I pulled up a chair, put down my supplies, and held her hand. I let her know I was there for her. "What's wrong?" I asked.

"I don't know," she replied, wiping her eyes, "I've just been here three times in the last month, and they can't figure out what is wrong with me." I listened and nodded. I didn't say anything. I just let her talk. Through her story I came to learn the real reason she was crying. She was scared she was going to find out something terrible like she was going to die and leave behind all the people she loved, including her children. She told me she had faith in God but could not feel His presence. As I listened to her, I felt compelled to remind her that when she was a child she would go to bed and sleep knowing all would be well, trusting that her parents would take care of everything when her parents may have been worried about things in their lives. Parents don't share their burdens with their children; yet often they carry many worries in their hearts. Parents may be worried that they will lose their jobs, or their home, or not know where the money is coming from to get groceries the next week. I told her this was a similar situation: Just like she trusted her parents so long ago and fell asleep without worry she had to trust that her God would take care of her now. She smiled and squeezed my hand. I gave her more tissues and proceeded to start her IV and hang the antibiotics. It had been over 30 minutes. I was not getting home on time for sure. I called the kids and said good night, finished up with my last tasks and charts, and went home. The next day when I saw my patient again, she was smiling. She grabbed my hands. "Thank you," she said, "your words helped me make it through the night; you don't know how much they helped me." She told me she wanted me to know this and was praying I would be her nurse again so that she could tell me just how important those words were to her so that I would never forget, and I haven't throughout all these years. The compassion we show and the words we say really do *matter* for the patient's experience.

Lynette's Experience

The year that I turned 39, I went in for my yearly well-women's exam with my gynecologist. I always schedule my yearly checkups near my birthday as a present to myself. Each year is a gift, and staying on top of my preventative care appointments is one way that I can take steps to give myself as many years with my family as possible. I knew that I was 1 year away from needing to get my first mammogram, and to be honest I was excited that I still had a whole year before I had to. As the exam progressed, my doctor felt something in my left breast that she wanted me to have checked, so I ended up not getting that extra year after all.

I went in, they did a diagnostic mammogram, and thankfully, despite what I had heard from other female family members in my life, they did not squish my breasts irreparably into a pancake shape, and it didn't hurt me at all. I was even more relieved after my diagnostic mammogram and ultrasound, as the images were clear. However, now I am on a yearly mammogram schedule, and each time I went in an area was found that needed to be reexamined, so the fearful feelings continued for me every time.

That brings me to this last year. I went in for my mammogram, and sure enough, a few days later I got the phone call that I needed to come in for more imaging. During the first phone call I was told that my left breast needed further imaging, and when I called back to schedule, I asked if I could speak with someone because it had been the left breast the last time. I had been told that once I had an image history of a few years, the images would be able to be compared, and perhaps I wouldn't need a full diagnostic each time, so when I called, I wanted to know if they had seen a change in the area on my left breast. They told me that the area that they wanted to look at this time was measuring a different depth than the area that they were measuring before, so I agreed to come in. Later that night, when I was looking in my chart, I saw that the order had been put in to look at my right breast, not the left. There was a note that the doctor made a transcription error and said left when he meant right, so it was the right breast that needed more images.

This made me even more nervous. I understand that mistakes can happen. As a mental health provider, I am familiar with healthcare-related, record-keeping software, and I know that when we amend a chart, we want to keep a record of the amending, so I was glad the explanation was added to the chart. I did have some additional questions, though. My left breast had a history of needing further images. Now we were talking about the right, and I knew a mistake had been made. Still, I wanted to know how we knew for certain that the mistake was made in transcription and not in reading the films. I wanted to be sure that the radiologist hadn't been looking at the left side and thinking it was the right instead of merely saying the wrong word. Again, I was okay with the mistake, but I wanted someone to help me understand how we knew where the mistake had taken place rather than just moving forward to only look at the right side.

If the mistake were in fact in reading the wrong image, then *maybe* there had been breast cancer growing in the left that we'd been overlooking for a while. I wanted to know how we knew that the right side was really the "right" side to look at. When I came in for the appointment, I asked if I could speak with the radiologist and ask some questions. You would have thought I was asking for a miracle; the radiologist was not used to speaking directly with patients, and that was made known to me, but she reluctantly agreed to come speak with me before we did any imaging. The first thing she did was let me know that she was not the radiologist who made the mistake. She said that the radiologist who did was not working that day, but that she had spoken to him. He felt bad about making the mistake, but mistakes do happen. I told her I appreciated her speaking with me. I assured her that I didn't fault anyone for the mistake, but I did want to know how we knew the mistake was with transcription and not with thinking he was looking at the right when it was the left. I asked if there was anything in the image that made it so they could tell it was my left or right breast. Was a shoulder also in the image or maybe one of my arms or some other internal structure that would help us know for certain that maybe the technician hadn't labeled the sides incorrectly when the images were taken, or was there some other way of knowing? The radiologist completely dismissed my fears. She literally said, "The error was with transcription. The other doctor graduated from Harvard. He is smart. He just made a mistake."

I felt completely unheard. I never once questioned the doctor's intelligence. I never once blamed him for his mistake. I wanted to know for certain that we weren't looking at the right side, when there may be something going on the left side. I told her that her answer was not comforting. I told her that her answer did not actually answer my question at all, and it felt very dismissive. She became defensive, and she finally put me on the spot and told me that if I didn't trust them at this hospital, then I could go elsewhere.

That is when the nurse spoke up. The nurse told the radiologist that she had images pulled up of each of my breasts ready to show me. She could show me how they knew which side was which. She said breast tissue is unique, like a fingerprint, and they could tell which side was which by comparing it to my images from previous years. She asked if I wanted to see the images, and she took the time to show me where the area was on the right that they were going to look at today.

I had gone from feeling completely condescended to and treated like an inconvenience to feeling seen. The nurse saw my fear. She listened to me. I was able to tell her that my dad died when I was 14, that I had children at home who I didn't want to leave any earlier than I had to, and that I had six close friends who had all been diagnosed with breast cancer in their 40s. She was able to see how I felt and that I needed to be listened to. She answered my legitimate questions and eased my fears. I was able to feel like a human with her. I was able to be vulnerable and tell her that with every mammogram for the last 4 years showing problems, I was beginning to feel like I was just playing a waiting game with cancer. I wondered when it was going to show up for me, and I was scared. I also had valid questions and deserved to be heard by someone who cared. This was my body and my health care, and I had a voice in it.

At the time of the mammogram appointment, we were in the infant stages of developing the idea for this textbook and had already been published on the topic of **motivational interviewing** for health care providers creating what I call a **sacred space** for our patients, but this example showed me exactly what it was like to experience each of the health care approaches that we outline in this book. The radiologist was very much the "expert," defending her colleague, when I wasn't even attacking him, by saying that he was smart. He was Harvard trained, and I should just trust it. The nurse, on the other hand, saw that I was a person, and I simply wanted to know that we had the right side. She took the time to show me scientifically how they knew it was the right side we needed to look at today. She still educated me, with permission, because I asked, and—and this is a big "and"—she allowed me to educate *her* on my experiences and my life. That is what we want to empower providers to do in their work moving forward. We want to show providers how to *listen*, how to engage, how to *be a guide*, and how to *empower* their patients instead of just being an expert in the room.

We give these two examples to illustrate what is important to the patient and why we as clinicians need to allow our patients the time to tell us about who they are. First, we must listen to *their* stories and let them *educate us* about what they are going through. Then we can begin to build an emotional connection to support them through some of the hardest changes and challenges they may be facing. This space we are calling "sacred" is a space where patients can be vulnerable, and we should honor this space by being present for them in that moment. The space we create with our patients should resemble the space we would want to be in with our provider and how we would like to be heard and honored.

Dr. Charon, a pioneer in the field of **narrative medicine**, spoke at a white coat ceremony for medical students and told them the importance of listening to their patients' stories. She told them that she used to ask a litany of questions to find out what was wrong. She has since changed her approach. Now she sits on her hands to keep her from writing and finds it more useful to invite them to tell her their story of what brought them here today. She gives them her full attention, sometimes with "mouth wide open" and listens. It is this *joining of forces* between the provider and the patient, truly understanding, or trying to, that builds on **empathy** and trust—both of which are a necessary component to the collaborative approach (Awdish & Berry, 2017).

Barriers to Effective Communication

Ineffective Listening

One barrier to effective communication is thinking you don't have time to listen. This is one of the most frequently cited complaints by providers about not taking the time to listen to their patients. But as Awdish and Berry (2017) point out, hurried care is not without a price. By not identifying the root cause of the problem the patient will continue to come back, requiring more testing until an answer is found, costing the healthcare system untold amounts of money and the patient untold amounts of frustration.

Example

A 46-year-old female patient comes in with complaints of passing out after every bowel movement with subsequent fatigue lasting all day, preventing her from being able to work. She is now terrified of having a bowel movement and is experiencing constipation. She has a strong family history of needing pacemaker placements, and an EKG reveals bradycardia down to 46 beats per minute in the office. A cardiologist referral is made; orders for an echocardiogram, stress test, and 30-day Holter monitor are nonrevealing. The patient is given a referral by the cardiologist to a gastroenterologist, who does an upper and lower endoscopy for no clear reason. Both are negative for finding a problem other than mild gastritis, for which patients are given a prescription for a proton pump inhibitor, and it is suggested that she might want to see a psychiatrist. Patient sees a psychiatrist who prescribes an antidepressant, which is called for as she is now very depressed. It has been over a year, and her symptoms have not improved; subsequently, she has lost her job. Her husband thinks it is all "in her head," and at this point she does too.

Finally, she goes back to her primary care provider's office, and it is suggested she see a different cardiologist, but this time the provider calls the cardiologist and explains the patients' symptoms and what work-up she has been through as well as their concerns. More tests are done, and an internal cardiac loop recorder is implanted. The long-awaited answer was soon found. The tracing shows she goes into a fine atrial flutter with her bowel movements. This is what was causing her to pass out and have profound fatigue for the rest of the day. She feels vindicated. She is not crazy. This is easily corrected with a cardiac ablation and for the first time in 2 long years she is symptom free.

Things to Think About

- Did the first cardiologist explore all options for a vasovagal response?
- Was a referral to gastroenterology needed?
- Was psychiatry the answer for her symptoms?
- Were her visits hurried?
- Did anyone take the time to *listen to* her story?

Defensiveness

Avoid at all costs becoming defensive about your care or recommendations, as this will do little to change the situation. You are not on trial, and if the patient is upset, listen to their concerns. Once you understand what their concerns are, you can address them in a way your patient can hear you.

Example

As illustrated in Lynette's story earlier in this chapter, the radiologist totally misread the situation and the concern. She became defensive and protective of the care that was being offered, feeling like she needed to point out that her colleague had gone to Harvard and was smart, when that is not what Lynette was questioning. If the nurse had not intervened, Lynette would have left the clinic more worried and felt totally dismissed. The nurse did *not* become defensive; she listened and determined what Lynette needed. She was able to show Lynette on the images of her breast how they could tell for sure which breast was which and which needed to be looked at that day, alleviating her fear. This allowed Lynette to feel like she could trust this individual, and she was able to share more of her story with her, transitioning the experience from feeling dismissed to feeling heard and validated.

Things to Think About

- Do I understand the patient's perspective?
- Am I taking this personally?
- How can I redirect this conversation to become more positive?

Health Literacy

Health literacy is another barrier in communication. We often use terms in medicine that are so common to us that we do not even think about it when we are talking to patients. According to the Milken Institute (Lopez et al., 2022), 88% of adults in the United States have some degree of health illiteracy that makes navigating the healthcare system difficult. It is important to realize that a person can be highly educated but still be illiterate when it comes to health care. Using simple terms instead of medical jargon as well as visual aids, apps, or prompts can be very helpful in explaining complicated medical conditions to any patient regardless of their educational status.

Example

Patient is a 52-year-old, male and has a doctorate in education. He has been diagnosed with atrial fibrillation, a cardiac arrhythmia that is characterized by disorderly electrical activity in the atria of his heart. Normally the sinoatrial node known as the pacemaker gives the electrical signal, but his heart has electrical impulses that override this impulse, causing erratic behavior, from which the ventricles are trying to respond. The result is an irregular rhythm that can be dangerous because it can cause clots to form, which can end up in the brain, causing a stroke. He is told he will need to take an anticoagulant for the rest of his life. He leaves feeling uncertain about his diagnosis and with a prescription in hand that he is not sure he wants to take.

A simpler explanation could have been accompanied by an app that you can download on your phone that shows the heart beating in normal sinus rhythm and the erratic electrical activity when the heart is in atrial fibrillation. Given this visual, the patient can understand why the heartbeat is irregular and not as strong as the provider explains how the electrical current works in the heart and why a blood thinner is needed to keep a clot from forming in the heart, which could cause a stroke. This approach may achieve much better results in terms of the patient taking the medication. Health literacy training is something all providers should engage in and is available at the Centers for Disease Control (CDC) for all providers at cdc.gov/health-literacy/php/find-training/get-training.html

Things to Think About

- Are you using simple words?
- Could a fifth grader understand you?
- How can you explain things in a way that your patient can relate to?
- What visual aids can you incorporate to help the patient visualize what you are saying?

Cultural Sensitivity and Diversity

There is no denying the disparities we have in healthcare with minority populations in all areas when we look at the statistics/feedback from patients regarding their health care experiences. Providers who do not exhibit **cultural sensitivity or diversity** will have barriers in communication with these groups. For each of these groups we have given some background and facts of that experience. Each group has reported explicit and **implicit bias** when they have attempted to seek health care by the providers and workers whose job it is to help them. We have also illustrated an example to help you *see through the eyes of their diversity*. Only by recognizing and seeing the bias can we hope to eliminate it and provide the best care possible to all patients no matter what their background is, their beliefs, the color of their skin, or the culture they grew up in. As you read through each scenario, ask yourself how you as a provider would react in each given situation.

LGBTQ+ Persons

Facts

According to the CDC (2024d), 33% of LGB students have been bullied in school, 48% have considered suicide, 63% have felt sad or hopeless, 23% have used illicit drugs, 22% have been forced to have sex, and 24% have misused prescription opioid. LGBTQ+ patients often report feeling misunderstood by providers and that providers are not trained in how to care for them; they feel they are victims of bias when trying to get health care, often causing them to delay treatment.

Example

Imagine that you are a lesbian female who is coming in for your well-woman check and the provider asks about your preferred birth control, assuming you are a heterosexual. Would you feel comfortable discussing this with them?

Autistic People

Facts

According to CDC (2025b), one in 36 children have been diagnosed with autism spectrum disorder, and this condition is reported four times more frequently in boys. Autistic patients and parents of autistic children often report failure of providers or health care workers in understanding the care they need to be given or report being the recipient of suboptimal care resulting in hesitation to seek health care treatment, leading to delays in care.

Example

Imagine being the mother of a 3-year-old boy who has autism. He has an earache, and you are worried about an ear infection, but you are even more worried about how the doctor's appointment will go. Will they approach your son in a way he will receive? Will it be a struggle? From previous experience you know how long your son can remember a bad experience, which can cause meltdowns and nightmares for many months to come. You wonder if they will understand and take cues from you, his primary caregiver, as to the best approach. What would be your approach in this situation?

Unhoused Persons

Facts

According to CDC (2024a), about 40% of unhoused people stay in unsheltered locations like a car or outside; the rest are in some type of emergency shelter. Due to congregate shelters, unhoused people are at greater risk for infectious and noninfectious diseases (CDC, 2024e).

Example

Imagine that you are being discharged from a hospital but have nowhere to go. There is no ride to call, and you have no money for the prescriptions they say you must have. You look outside and see it has become colder. The nurse tells you about the medicine you know you cannot afford and that you must follow up with an appointment at the clinic in 1 week, but you have no idea how you will get there. You wonder, if you can't do these things will you be considered "noncompliant" with their medical plan?

- What resources could you provide for this patient?
- Do you have access to a social worker?

See the Neighborhood Navigator tool (https://www.aafp.org/family-physician/patient-care/the-everyone-project/neighborhood-navigator.html).

Immigrants

Facts

Immigrants face many healthcare disparities. Not only are they trying to adjust to a new country, but many do not have medical insurance. Language may also be a barrier, workplace conditions may be poor, and they may have income inequality and lack education (CDC, 2025a).

Example

Imagine that you have immigrated to the United States. You struggle with the language, and one of your children becomes ill. You do not have much money and have no medical insurance. Where will you go to get help? You can go to the emergency room, but what about follow-up care if you need it? How much more complicated would this situation be if you were undocumented? Imagine how you would feel if you overheard a conversation from healthcare workers about illegal immigrants and healthcare?

- What resources could you give this patient for follow-up care?
- How will you address your own bias?

Marginalized Income or Social Class

Facts

People from lower socioeconomic status are subject to higher rates of mental illness, chronic disease, higher mortality, and lower life expectancy (Singh & Siahpush, 2006).

Example

Imagine being a diabetic patient with only Social Security to live on. You struggle to pay your rent and get your medicine, and the provider is talking about adding more fresh fruits and vegetables to your diet. The nearest big grocery store is over 30 miles away, and you do not have transportation, so you get all your food at the local one, which has much higher prices. You think to yourself, "If they only knew all you could afford to eat all week is the big pot of spaghetti you make on Sunday." You don't say anything because you don't really feel they will understand.

- Do you take into consideration the ability to get groceries when you are talking to a patient who needs to improve their diet?
- How will you bring this up in a sensitive way?
- Are you aware of resources in your area you could refer patients to?

Black, Indigenous, and People of Color

Facts

According to a study by Macias-Konstantopoulos et al. (2023), there is overwhelming evidence that points to an "inextricable link" between race and health care disparities. The study looked at communicable diseases, noncommunicable conditions, and injuries.

Example

Imagine you are the mother of a teenage Black girl who has been suffering from headaches, and they find that her blood pressure is very elevated (220/110), causing her to miss multiple days of school. You have taken her to the pediatrician and the urgent care multiple times, and they keep giving you medicine for her blood pressure and saying she has high blood pressure because of her race, but you think to yourself, "Isn't it odd that she is so young with such high blood pressure? Why are the pills they are giving you not working? Why are they not sending you to a specialist?" How would you handle this situation?

Marginalized Religious Groups

Facts

People who belong to marginalized religions have reported disparities in healthcare because providers do not understand their beliefs: Jewish people, Muslims, Seventh-day Adventists, Jehovah's Witnesses, practitioners of Indigenous spiritual traditions, and many others. Spirituality is tied to many decisions that could impact medical decisions.

Example

You are a Muslim woman, and you are coming for your postnatal exam. You thought you would be seeing a woman doctor but are being seen by the male doctor in the office. This is not allowed in your religion. What are you going to do? Will he understand if you request a female provider? (Swihart et al., 2023)

- How would you react?
- How will you become aware of a patient's different beliefs that you need to be sensitive to?

People in Larger Bodies

Facts

Often people who are overweight or obese may not seek health care because of perceived provider bias (Fruh et al., 2016). Body mass index (BMI) is a metric we measure at each visit, which can cause undue stress on an individual coming in for an acute problem. We might ask ourselves, "If that is something we need to do on every visit for every problem even when it has nothing to do with weight?"

Example

Imagine being overweight from a medical condition that you cannot control, but every time you come to the doctor's office the office staff makes you feel awful about your weight. Many times, you come to the office for other complaints that have nothing to do with your weight, but you still have to stand on the scale and have the conversation with the provider about weight loss. How would that make you feel? What will your policy be with weight on every visit? Should it be only well-being unless you are doing a weight management visit?

Ageism

Facts

Ageism is real. Older adults spend on average 21 days a year on medical visits and often experience people speaking loudly to them, assuming that they cannot hear or understand what is being said or talking to their children about their health care when they are very capable of speaking for themselves (Milne-Tyte, 2024).

Example

Imagine being older in the hospital and looking unkempt because you are sick. The hospital staff doesn't listen to you. They talk over you, speak louder, and talk to your family in regard to you as if you are not there. You are still a vibrant person very capable of taking care of yourself and your affairs. In fact, you still work full-time and run a business. How would that make you feel?

- How will you interact with older patients?
- What if they are beginning to become forgetful?

Prisoners

Facts

The incarceration rate is the highest in the world in the United States. Many of the inmates come from socioeconomically disadvantaged communities and are from people in minority groups. They have higher rates of tuberculosis and HIV, hepatitis, diabetes, and mental health (Alsan et al., 2023). They have health care but often must wait a long time to get an appointment, and they have a copay that can be as high as a month's wages, just to see a provider who often in their opinion gives substandard care.

Example

Imagine being an inmate during the initial phases of the COVID-19 pandemic. There is not enough personal protective equipment, there are not enough medical personnel, and you live in a crowded environment. You find out the person in the cell next to you has COVID and is coughing. How do you feel? Will the system be able to take care of you if you get sick?

- Are you aware of the screening tests you might want to offer?
- How will you approach asking them if they would like various screening tests?

People Who Are HIV Positive

Facts

According to the CDC (2024c), 37,981 people in 2022 were told they had HIV, and 38% of these people were Black/African Americans, 32% Hispanic/Latino, and 24% White. Stigma and discrimination still surround the diagnosis of HIV, preventing many people from finding out their HIV status or seeking treatment.

Example

Imagine what it would be like to hear the words "you are HIV positive." What would be your initial thoughts? How would this impact your life, your dreams, those close to you? The next time you have your blood drawn would you feel compelled to tell the person drawing your blood your HIV status? Would you worry about how providers might treat you or ask you the dreaded question on how you got it? Would you feel like an outcast even though treatment options have become much more effective and work to destigmatize the disease has grown over the years, or would you still feel like hiding the truth?

- How will you handle screening for HIV and that conversation?
- How will you handle screening for Prep (HIV prophylaxis?)

Mental Health Disorders

Facts

In many communities people still do not recognize mental health conditions as legitimate disorders. They continue to blame and shame those with conditions like anxiety and depression, as though the person caused it themselves or as if they have the power to control the symptoms completely on their own. The stigmatization of mental disorders is a significant barrier to receiving care (Ahad et al., 2023).

Example

Imagine suffering from depression for a long time but not being able to talk to anyone about it because in your family they do not talk about mental illness. You finally get the courage to bring up the subject with your provider. What would you hope for in response from the provider? What would be going through your mind?

- What screening recommendations will you use for depression and anxiety?
- Do you have a plan if they screen positive to formally diagnose them?
- Do you have resources for them to go to for further care?
- Are you comfortable starting them on medications?

Pregnant Teens

Facts

U.S. teen birth rates are declining, but according to the CDC (2024b) they are still higher than many other high-income countries. From 1991 to 2021, the U.S. teen birth rate per 1,000 for girls aged 15–19 has decreased 78%, with evidence pointing to abstinence and birth control.

Example

Imagine you are 15 years old looking down at a home pregnancy test that is positive. What would be going through your mind? How would your life change as soon as everyone knows? What would you think about when you saw the doctor for the first time? Would you feel judged—even years later as an older woman when people begin that calculation and you see in their eyes when they find out how old your child is and realize your age? Will those thoughts ever go away, or will you just get used to them?

- How will you protect a teen's anonymity if they come to you for a visit but are using their parents' insurance? (Parents get a statement of visits and tests run if it is their insurance.)
- Do you know where the local health clinics are to refer them to in your area?

People With Substance Use Disorders

Facts

Substance use disorder (SUD) is prevalent in the United States, with data showing that nearly 50 million Americans have experienced it in the last year. Mental illness often occurs with SUD but is rarely treated together in health care settings. Heroin use is increasing across *all* income levels.

Example

You are a 53-year-old female coming in to see your nurse practitioner for help with stomach pain that has been worsening over the last few weeks. You have a history of alcohol dependence. You've cut back on your drinking, but you haven't stopped completely. Do you fear that your provider will focus solely on the alcohol use and dismiss everything else, insisting that nothing can be done to help you until you are completely "sober"? Or are you able to have hope, knowing that your provider listens and will work to help you address both issues?

- How will you help your patients who have end-stage liver disease related to alcohol abuse?
- Liver transplants can only be done if a patient is 6 months sober. How will you discuss this with your patients?
- How will you help patients who relapse with their drug of choice?

Language Barriers

Finally, language can be a barrier to effective communication. In America, we now have one in five households that speak a different language other than English. Language barriers pose many problems, from understanding what the diagnosis entails to how to take medication or follow directions for a test. Misunderstanding can lead to adverse health events, with one study showing that detectable adverse events happened 49% of the time and moderate temporary harm occurred 47% of the time (Deering, 2023). Having bilingual professionals is one way to combat this problem, or utilize an approved medical interpreting service. Electronic medical records (EMRs) that can print patient summaries in multiple languages are also very beneficial. Multicultural training can be obtained through the U.S. Department of Health and Human Services as an e-learning product (thinkculturalhealth.hhs.gov/nursing/).

Example

Patient is 48 years old and only speaks Spanish. He comes to the office with pain in the right kidney area. A kidney stone is suspected, and he is sent for a CT of his abdomen. It comes back showing a large irregular mass, which is highly suspicious for malignancy. He has always come to the office with an interpreter from his family, but this time we need a medical interpreter to make sure he understands what we found and what the next steps are. Through the help of the medical interpreter, we are assured he understands his diagnosis and what his options are. He has ultimately decided to go back to his home country for treatment.

- Why did they need to use a reliable medical interpreter?
- Why do you feel he decided to go back to his home country for treatment?

We have taken time to give you facts about each of these groups and an example of what it would feel like to walk in their shoes. These stories are about real people who exist in the files of our memory. Only through understanding a patient's story and seeing the world as they see it can we hope to build upon that relationship of trust that is so important in the patient-provider relationship.

The Importance of Empathy and Trust

It has been said, "Empathy is the medicine the world needs," and there is truth to that. Carl Rogers coined the term "empathic listening" because he felt that psychoanalysts did too much of the talking and not enough of the listening at the time. Rogers believed that if a patient was able to feel truly listened to and understood, he could create an environment where patients could make positive changes in their lives (Guenther, 2022). Rogers believed that creating a space where empathy was offered, and therapeutic trust could be established, was essential for positive change. He felt this empathic, trusting relationship needed to happen first, and until it did change would not take place. Rogers also believed that change came from *within the patient, not from within the therapist.* He viewed the patient, not the provider, as the expert. This is what Rogers meant by person-centered or humanistic psychology.

This does not mean that the provider does not have expertise or information to share with patients based on lab work and specific health conditions, but it does mean that the patient decides what happens next. One of the main things that providers can do to set the stage for work with patients in this way is to offer empathic listening, to take the time to truly understand what is being said, not just to take in the words. Empathic listening involves the following

- *Be present:* Set aside your own agenda and focus on what the patient is saying. When we spend more time focusing on what we are going to say next, we miss the message that the patient is communicating to us.
- *Pay attention to nonverbal cues:* Listen not only for words but to everything that the patient conveys. We know that nonverbals cues send a stronger message than what the person is saying, so listen for those too. What body language is the person displaying? Do they appear to be comfortable and engaged, or are they reluctant, confused, angry, or fearful?
- *Suspend judgment:* Keep an open mind. Notice our internal biases and set those aside. Don't make statements that are critical or judgmental. Be curious. Every message that the patient sends gives us information about where they are. We don't need to judge it. We need to take it in as useful data that can help us gain a clearer picture of the needs of our patients.
- *Validate the emotions and experiences of patients:* Use statements like, "I can see why you would feel that way" or "That sounds really hard." Don't minimize or try to put a positive spin on what the person is sharing with you.

- *Offer paraphrases and summaries of information shared:* This can look like repeating a small portion of what was said or offering a summary of it in your own words. This will give the patient the chance to see that you understood and will allow them the opportunity to correct you if you misinterpreted something.
- *Don't rush to solutions:* Focus on being a supportive listener first. After you have demonstrated that you understand and that you care, you will build trust and have the foundation of empathy and trust needed to develop solutions together.

The most frequent complaint in healthcare is that patients have not felt listened to (King, 2022). We need to change that. Patients are often at their most vulnerable state when at the hospital or meeting with their doctor. Developing empathic listening skills can ease fears and create a more collaborative space for patients and providers.

To illustrate the fact that empathy and compassion really matter, let's look at a study conducted by Johns Hopkins University regarding HIV patients being compliant with their treatment (Beach et al., 2006). HIV has come a long way from being considered a death sentence and is now a very well-controlled chronic disease with compliance to antiviral drug therapy. It is important for patients to take the medication exactly as prescribed. Johns Hopkins wanted to know if a compassionate connection between the patient and the provider could make a difference. The sample size was 1,700 patients with HIV. The study asked the participants to respond to the yes or no question "Does your HIV provider really know you as a person?" They looked for an association between the three variables: (a) being known as a person by the provider, (b) HIV viral load, (c) medication adherence. In the patients who felt known as a person by the provider, they had 33% higher odds of being compliant with medication adherence and 20% higher odds of having no detectable viral load in their blood. These results are astounding and *so* simple to enact (Beach et al., 2006). Just knowing that if your patients feel you know them as a person and care can cause this much of an increase in positive results should motivate all of us to do better.

Patient Involvement in Care Decisions

Historically, medical paternalism was the model held for centuries based on the belief that physicians were experts in medical matters, and their main duty was to promote the patient's welfare. Providers were the experts and held the keys to necessary testing, procedures, and medication that patients needed. Providers developed medical health care plans based on their assessment and diagnosis that were in the patients' best interests. The patient's health status was deemed the provider's responsibility. If patients did not follow the plan they were considered "noncompliant."

Since the 1950s we have seen a shift to emphasizing patients' rights and the need for a more collaborative approach. Patient-centered care or **shared decision-making** have become the new model. In this model providers are still the experts with medical knowledge and background, but patients are consulted regarding their health care plan to take into consideration their customs, beliefs, and preferences. The hope is if patients are involved in the planning process of their health care and it is more personalized, they will be more compliant with the recommendations, and we will see better health care outcomes.

Today, with the birth of technology and access to medical information, direct patient testing, and tracking devices, patients can become more involved in their health care than ever before. Today, when a patient has a problem, they get on the internet and research it completely. They have access to direct-to-consumer testing and genetic profiles, and they can track multiple aspects of their health (Kilbride & Joffe, 2018). The provider is now seen more in consultation as we move to a more patient-driven model of healthcare. This model focuses more on codiagnosing and cocare among providers, patients and others. The access to this type of information is empowering patients *to not only be active in their health care plan but to drive it* (Swan, 2009). Providers are still responsible for bringing to the table expertise and appropriateness for testing or medication management but are not seen as the one responsible for the outcomes as much as the patient is. This model may prove to be the one that is the most useful in not only compliance with a medical plan but improved medical outcomes.

KEY POINTS

- Learn to listen to and hear the patient's story.
- Understand your biases and the judgments you bring with you.
- Speak in simple terms.
- Recognize patients as the experts in the room when it comes to their own identities and lived experiences.
- Allow them to educate you about what they need.
- See them as a person.
- Find out what is most important for them to talk about with you today.

QUESTIONS FOR REFLECTION

- What type of provider do you want to be?
- Do you have a good understanding of the patients you will be treating?
- What is your understanding of a good **patient experience** with a provider?
- Which model of healthcare have you grown up with?

- Can you think of a provider you really liked or would like to be like?
- Can you think of a provider you really would not want to be like?

SUGGESTED ACTIVITIES

1. Write about what type of provider you want to be prior to reading the chapter and then reflect on that letter after the reading and see if anything you read altered your thoughts.
2. Pair up in teams of two to four and discuss your experiences with healthcare that were good and those that were bad. Identify the conditions that were different in each scenario. Here are some suggested questions you might want to explore.
   a. What made the experience good?
   b. What made the experience bad?
   c. Did you feel heard?
   d. Did you have a voice in your care?
   e. Were your questions answered?
3. Have students develop an infographic regarding a marginalized group from a patient perspective. Include a YouTube video from a person in this diversity category, explaining what their healthcare experience was like.
4. Do a health literacy assignment in which a student explains a highly complicated health care issue to a patient and checks the grade level at which they explain it. Have students make revisions until they have explained it at a fifth grade reading level. Have them include visuals or apps they would incorporate into the patient teaching.

References

Ahad, A. A., Sanchez-Gonzalez, M., & Junquera, P. (2023). Understanding and addressing mental health stigma across cultures for improving psychiatric care: A narrative review. *Cureus, 15(5), e39549.* https://doi.org/10.7759/cureus.39549

Alsan, M., Yang, C. S., Jolin, J. R., Tu, L., & Rich, J. D. (2023). Health care in U.S. correctional facilities—A limited and threatened constitutional right. *New England Journal of Medicine, 388*(9), 847–852. https://doi.org/10.1056/nejmms2211252

Awdish, R. L., & Berry, L. L. O. (2017, October 9). *Making time to really listen to your patients. Harvard Business Review.* https://hbr.org/2017/10/making-time-to-really-listen-to-your-patients

Beach, M. C., Keruly, J., & Moore, R. D. (2006). Is the quality of the patient-provider relationship associated with better adherence and health outcomes for patients with HIV? *Journal of General Internal Medicine, 21*(6). https://doi.org/10.1111/j.1525-1497.2006.00399_1.x

Centers for Disease Control and Prevention. (2024a, October 15). *About homelessness and health.* https://www.cdc.gov/homelessness-and-health/about/index.html#:~:text=Around%2040%25%20of%20people%20experiencing%20homelessness%20live%20in,have%20higher%20rates%20of%20homelessness.%20Homelessness%20and%20health

Centers for Disease Control and Prevention. (2024b, May15).*About teen pregnancy.* https://www.cdc.gov/reproductive-health/teen-pregnancy/index.html

Centers for Disease Control and Prevention. (2024c, June 27). *Fast facts: HIV in the US by race and ethnicity.* https://www.cdc.gov/hiv/data-research/facts-stats/race-ethnicity.html

Centers for Disease Control and Prevention. (2024d, November 29). *Health disparities among LGBTQ youth.* https://www.cdc.gov/healthy-youth/lgbtq-youth/health-disparities-among-lgbtq-youth.html?CDC_AAref_Val=https://www.cdc.gov/healthyyouth/disparities/health-disparities-among-lgbtq-youth.htm

Centers for Disease Control and Prevention. (2025a, January 31). *About immigrant and refugee health.* https://www.cdc.gov/immigrant-refugee-health/about/index.html#:~:text=Immigrants%2C%20refugees%2C%20and%20migrants%2C%20especially%20if%20recently%20resettled,healthcare%20workplace%20conditions%20education%20income%20and%20wealth%20gap

Centers for Disease Control and Prevention. (2025b, May 27). *Data and statistics on autism spectrum disorder.* https://www.cdc.gov/autism/data-research/index.html

Deering, M. (2023, September 29). *Addressing language barriers in healthcare.* Nurse Journal. https://nursejournal.org/articles/language-barriers-in-healthcare/

Fruh, S. M., Nadglowski, J., Hall, H. R., Davis, S. L., Crook, E. D., & Zlomke, K. (2016). Obesity stigma and bias. *The Journal for Nurse Practitioners, 12*(7), 425–432. https://doi.org/10.1016/j.nurpra.2016.05.013

Guenther, K. (2022). "Umm, mm'h, yeah": Carl Rogers, phonographic recordings, and the making of therapeutic listening. *History of Psychology, 25*(3), 191–https://doi.org/10.1037/hop0000216

Kilbride, M. K., & Joffe, S. (2018). The new age of patient autonomy. *JAMA, 320*(19), 1973–1974. https://doi.org/10.1001/jama.2018.14382

King, G. (2022). Central yet overlooked: Engaged and person-centered listening and healthcare conversations. *Disability and Rehabilitation, 44*(24), 7664–7676. https://doi.org/10.1080/09638288.2021.1982026

Lopez, C., Kim, B., & Sacks, K. (2022). *Health literacy in the United States: Enhancing assessments and reducing disparities.* Milken Institute. https://milkeninstitute.org/sites/default/files/2022-05/Health_Literacy_United_States_Final_Report.pdf

Macias-Konstantopoulos, W. L., Collins, K. A., Diaz, R., Duber, H. C., Edwards, C. D., Hsu, A. P., Ranney, M. L., Riviello, R. J., Wettstein, Z. S., & Sachs, C. J. (2023). Race, healthcare, and health disparities: A critical review and recommendations for advancing health equity. *Western Journal of Emergency Medicine, 24*(5). https://doi.org/10.5811/westjem.58408

Milne-Tyte, A. (2024, March 7). *Ageism in health care is more common than you might think, and it can harm people.* NPR. https://www.npr.org/sections/health-shots/2024/03/07/1236371376/bias-ageism-older-adults-geriatrics

Shute, D. A. (2019). Motivational interviewing: Benefits and advice for busy physicians. *Contemporary OB/GYN, 60*(10), 38–40. https://www.contemporaryobgyn.net/view/motivational-interviewing-benefits-and-advice-busy-physicians

Singh, G. K., & Siahpush, M. (2006). Widening socioeconomic inequalities in us life expectancy, 1980–2000. *International Journal of Epidemiology, 35*(4), 969–979. https://doi.org/10.1093/ije/dyl083

Swan, M. (2009). Emerging patient-driven health care models: An examination of health social networks, consumer personalized medicine and quantified self-tracking. *International Journal of Environmental Research and Public Health, 6*(2), 492–525. https://doi.org/10.3390/ijerph6020492

Swihart, D. L., Yarrarapu, S. S., & Martin, R. L. (2023). *Cultural religious competence in clinical practice*. StatPearls. http://europepmc.org/books/NBK493216

Chapter 2

The Paternalistic or Expert Approach to Patient Care

In nothing do men more nearly approach the gods than in giving health to men.

—Cicero

In this chapter we will look at how medical care is changing and how the traditional medical model, or expert approach, developed throughout history. In times past, the provider held the keys to medical knowledge, testing, and medications. Today the patients are much more involved due to access to medical information thanks to the internet. Today, patients often thoroughly research a subject prior to coming in to see the provider. Also, patients have access to direct-to-consumer testing and can get results for pregnancy, sexually transmitted diseases, or general wellness panels from various groups and labs on their own. This evolution has prompted a reevaluation of the traditional medical model to a more patient-driven approach. Health care providers are urged to incorporate greater collaboration with their patients and shared decision-making, blending medical expertise with patient engagement, ultimately redefining the roles of both provider and patient in the quest for optimal health outcomes that are driven more by the patient.

OBJECTIVES

- Students will be able to define the medical model.
- Students will be able to describe the core competencies in education for various providers such as medical doctor (MD), doctor of osteopathy (DO), and physician assistant (PA).

- Students will be able to compare the difference between the traditional medical model and a more patient-driven approach.

KEY TERMS AND DEFINITIONS

- **Expert approach:** The provider assumes the role of an authority figure, making decisions on behalf of the patient without considering the patient's preferences or input, grounded in the belief that the provider knows what is best because they are the expert in the field.
- **Hippocratic oath:** An ethical pledge taken by medical professionals emphasizing beneficence (acting in the patient's best interest), nonmaleficence (doing no harm), confidentiality, and ethical responsibility in the practice of medicine.
- **Medical doctors (MDs):** Providers trained in the traditional medical model, focusing on evidence-based diagnosis and treatment of diseases, with education, including premedical undergraduate studies, medical school, and residency training.
- **Doctors of osteopathy (DOs):** Providers trained similarly to MDs but involving manipulative maneuvers with an emphasis on the interconnection of the mind, body, and spirit.
- **Physician Assistants (PAs):** Individuals who have received a master's degree involving learning the medical model. They practice under the supervision of MDs or DOs and are trained to provide medical care, including diagnosing illnesses, prescribing medications, and performing procedures, with a focus on patient-centered care.

The Medical Model

To understand the medical model of healthcare, we need to go back to the origins of medicine. Hippocrates, often referred to as the *father of medicine,* had a much different view on the patient-provider relationship than what is held today. Prior to Hippocrates, people who were ill attended temples and appealed to the gods for help with their illness. Priests and priestesses said prayers and incantations for the sick, but Hippocrates began to study illness in a different way. He taught a systematic way of looking at illness that in many ways persists today. Emphasis was placed on obtaining an accurate history, doing a thorough physical exam, observing, and recording signs and symptoms, classifying diseases, and recording what works and what does not work (Cushing, 1999). This model can be seen in the documentation of the history and physical exam (Table 2.1).

Table 2.1 **Medical Model**

Chief Complaint	"I have a sore throat."
History of the Present Illness (onset, location, duration, characteristics, aggravating factors, relieving factors, time, and severity [OLDCARTS])	The patient presents with a 3-day history of a sore throat. The patient states it feels like they are "swallowing needles" and reports having a low-grade fever with chills for the past 24 hours. The patient denies having a runny nose. They work in a school, so they are around children who are sick. Ibuprofen seems to help, as well as honey lemon tea. Eating and drinking make it worse. They rate their pain level an 8 out of 10.
Past Medical History	Hypertension
Past Surgical History	Gallbladder removed 3 years ago
Family History	Father has coronary heart disease; mother has hypertension and diabetes
Social History	Does not smoke, drinks only socially
Allergies	Penicillin
Current Medications	Valsartan 160mg
Review of Systems (Subjective Data)	General: C/o chills and fever HEENT: C/o sore throat, states it feels like swallowing pins and needles. Lungs: Denies cough Heart: Denies chest pain Abdomen: Denies nausea/ vomiting, or diarrhea Skin: Denies rash
Physical Exam (Objective Data)	General: Alert and well appearing HEENT: TMs pearly gray bilaterally, tonsils with erythema and exudate, 3+, no nasal drainage noted
Labs	Strep rapid (+)

Radiology	None
Other tests	None
Assessment/Diagnosis	Group A streptococcal throat infection
Plan	Amoxicillin 500mg BID × 10 days; Tylenol for fever, RTC if no improvement in 2–3 days; warm saltwater gargles, honey lemon tea as needed

We classify disease according to the International Classification of Diseases (ICD) and procedural codes with the Current Procedural Terminology (CPT). We also have many different scientific resources that are grounded in evidence to help providers know the best work-up to do as well as the most up-to-date treatment options, far surpassing anything that Hippocrates ever dreamed of. Back in the days of Hippocrates, medicine was not regulated. Some providers were legitimate, but others were considered opportunists. The **Hippocratic oath** was instituted to establish a clear framework for practicing medicine in an *ethical manner*. The goal was to elevate the practice of medicine to a respected profession based on knowledge, skills, and ethical responsibility. We have included copies of both the classic and revised Hippocratic oath for your review.

> *Classic Hippocratic Oath*[1]
> I swear by Apollo the physician, and Aesculapius the surgeon, likewise Hygeia and Panacea, and call all the gods and goddesses to witness, that I will observe and keep this underwritten oath, to the utmost of my power and judgment.
>
> I will reverence my master who taught me the art. Equally with my parents, will I allow him things necessary for his support, and will consider his sons as brothers. I will teach them my art without reward or agreement; and I will impart all my acquirement, instructions, and whatever I know, to my master's children, as to my own; and likewise, to all my pupils, who shall bind and tie themselves by a professional oath, but to none else.
>
> With regard to healing the sick, I will devise and order for them the best diet, according to my judgment and means; and I will take care that they suffer no hurt or damage.

1. Hippocrates, "Classic Hippocratic Oath," trans. W.H.S. Jones, 1923.

Nor shall any man's entreaty prevail upon me to administer poison to anyone; neither will I counsel any man to do so. Moreover, I will give no sort of medicine to any pregnant woman, with a view to destroy the child.

Further, I will comport myself and use my knowledge in a godly manner. I will not cut for the stone but will commit that affair entirely to the surgeons. Whatsoever house I may enter, my visit shall be for the convenience and advantage of the patient; and I will willingly refrain from doing any injury or wrong from falsehood, and (in an especial manner) from acts of an amorous nature, whatever may be the rank of those who it may be my duty to cure, whether mistress or servant, bond or free.

Whatever, in the course of my practice, I may see or hear (even when not invited), whatever I may happen to obtain knowledge of, if it be not proper to repeat it, I will keep sacred and secret within my own breast.

If I faithfully observe this oath, may I thrive and prosper in my fortune and profession, and live in the estimation of posterity; or on breach thereof, may the reverse be my fate! (Narsaria, 2015)

Medical students today, upon graduation, still take upon themselves a revised version of this oath by Dr. Louis Lasagna, academic dean at Tufts University School of Medicine (1964):

Revised Hippocratic Oath[2]
I swear to fulfill, to the best of my ability and judgment, this covenant:

I will respect the hard-won scientific gains of those physicians in whose steps I walk, and gladly share such knowledge as is mine with those who are to follow.

I will apply, for the benefit of the sick, all measures [that] are required, avoiding those twin traps of overtreatment and therapeutic nihilism.

I will remember that there is art to medicine as well as science, and that warmth, sympathy, and understanding may outweigh the surgeon's knife or the chemist's drug.

I will not be ashamed to say "I know not," nor will I fail to call in my colleagues when the skills of another are needed for a patient's recovery.

I will respect the privacy of my patients, for their problems are not disclosed to me that the world may know.

2. Louis Lasagna, "Modern Hippocratic Oath," 1964.

> Most especially must I tread with care in matters of life and death. If it is given me to save a life, all thanks. But it may also be within my power to take a life; this awesome responsibility must be faced with great humbleness and awareness of my own frailty.
>
> Above all, I must not play at God. I will remember that I do not treat a fever chart, a cancerous growth, but a sick human being, whose illness may affect the person's family and economic stability. My responsibility includes these related problems if I am to care adequately for the sick.
>
> I will prevent disease whenever I can, for prevention is preferable to cure. I will remember that I remain a member of society, with special obligations to all my fellow human beings, those sound of mind and body as well as the infirm. If I do not violate this oath, may I enjoy life and art, respected while I live and remembered with affection thereafter. May I always act so as to preserve the finest traditions of my calling and may I long experience the joy of healing those who seek my help. (Narsaria, 2015)

The main components of this oath include practicing in an ethical manner, practicing beneficence (act in the patients' best interests) and nonmaleficence (to do no harm), maintaining patient confidentiality, and not practicing in a harmful manner. During ancient times the average person had no access to medical information or training and was solely dependent on the physician to tell them the best course of action. The doctor was considered the expert in the matter, and they developed health care plans for the patient that they were expected to follow. Notice in both versions of the Hippocratic oath the health of the patient is the responsibility of the *provider*.

Doctors were elevated in some cultures to almost a god-like status, with patients not feeling as though they could question their authority. In the 1970s, for example, from my personal experience, when a doctor came into the hospital ward to see patients, nurses would give them their seats and assist them in making rounds. As a patient when you went to see the doctor, they were considered the expert and would give you their medical advice on how you should proceed. This paternalistic pattern did not take into consideration patient preferences as the advice given was grounded in science and considered to be in the patient's best interest. This attitude is still evidenced today with providers being given special privileges such as premium parking spots, free meals, and lounges to do their work uninterrupted while other health care workers do not enjoy such perks.

Patients who do not follow the advice of a provider, such as smoking or alcohol cessation, losing weight, or getting immunizations, are considered *noncompliant* and, in some cases, discharged from practice unless they conform to the recommendations. In theory, it seems reasonable to think that the paternalistic model works because providers are experts in the human body and disease, and if patients followed their advice they will be healthier. However, this approach rarely works. Ask any parent of a teenager and you will see this viewpoint is fraught with error. It is human nature to push back on or reject something that we are *told to do*, especially when we feel we do not have a choice (Berger & Villaume, 2020). We are hard-wired to want our free agency to make decisions even in matters for which we may not be the expert. Patient-centered care grew out of a need to get buy-in from patients to increase compliance to get better health care outcomes, but this has not been enough; we may need to take it one step further.

Patient-Centered Care

Patient-centered care began to be talked about in the 1950s, but did not really gain traction until 2001 with the Institute of Medicine's release of its seminal report, *Crossing the Quality Chasm: A New Health System for the 21st Century* (Cliff, 2012). Given the changing dynamics of an ageing population, coupled with medical information that can be found on the internet, patients were no longer in the dark. They were informed, although sometimes with misinformation, but they still wanted to be involved in the decision-making process.

Medicine was also changing from individual private practices to joining health care groups that were managed for efficiency. Health maintenance organizations (HMOs) and preferred provider organizations (PPOs) were the new model. The focus became on involving the patient and the family in the plan of care for better outcomes. The thought was if we considered what the patient's preferences were and took into consideration their culture and beliefs along with family support, we could develop a plan for their health that was more palatable to the patient and thus the patient would be more compliant, leading to improved outcomes. Although this is a much better plan than the paternalistic or expert model it is still provider driven *not* patient driven care. Let's consider the **expert approach** and the patient-centered approach.

Expert (Paternalistic) Approach

Following is an example of a provider-patient interaction that utilizes the expert or paternalistic approach:

> Provider: After reviewing your chest X-rays, it looks like you have emphysema of the lungs, and you will need to quit smoking.
>
> Patient: I'm not sure I can do that.
>
> Provider: If you do not quit smoking, you will end up on oxygen and may well die early from your disease.

Patient-Centered Approach

Following is an example of a provider-patient interaction that utilizes the patient-centered approach:

> Provider: After reviewing your chest X-rays, it looks like you have emphysema of the lungs, and you will need to quit smoking.
>
> Patient: I'm not sure I can do that.
>
> Provider: You could use nicotine patches or medication to cut down your desire to smoke. Which method do you feel would work for you? Do you have anyone who could support you in your efforts at home?

As you can see from both approaches, the patient is *still* being told they must quit smoking. In both cases the patient says they are not sure they can. They may not even want to, and that fact is not even considered in either approach. In the patient-centered approach, they are given some choices on how they can quit smoking, but it is still clear that they must stop smoking. If they choose not to quit smoking, they are deemed noncompliant to their care plan.

Education of Providers

Let's turn our attention to how different health care providers are trained in school by looking at the competencies that are required by the credentialing bodies. Competencies are components that credentialing bodies consider essential for a student to graduate. Pay attention to the different models of education and where the focus of learning is spent. We will look at three different models: **doctor of medicine (MD)**, **doctor of osteopathy (DO)**, and **physician assistant (PA)**. Starting with the MD, the credentialing body is the American Academy Medical Certification (AAMC). With this degree, a student must complete a 4-year undergraduate degree in premed with a focus on the sciences to apply for medical school. There are 17 competencies they must address before applying to medical school, three of which have to do with communication. They must demonstrate empathy and compassion, specifically understanding the patients' perspective. They must possess interpersonal and communication skills, which include active listening, listening to understand, and recognizing personal communication barriers (AAMC, n.d.b)

Once in medical school, the focus is on learning the medical model, with diagnosis and treatment at the forefront. They do include communication skills such as being able to counsel and educate patients and their families, as well as shared decision-making, effective communication, and being able to demonstrate sensitivity as well as being able to understand human emotions (Englander et al., 2013). After graduation from medical school there are 13 core activities that an applicant must have to enter residency, none of which involve communication with patients or their families (Table 2.2; AAMC, n.d.a.).

Table 2.2 **Residency Requirements**

1.	Gather a history and perform a physical exam.
2.	Prioritize a differential diagnosis following a clinical encounter.
3.	Recommend and interpret common diagnostic and screening tests.
4.	Enter and discuss orders and prescriptions.
5.	Document a clinical encounter in the patient record.
6.	Provide an oral presentation of a clinical encounter.
7.	Form clinical questions and retrieve evidence to advance patient care.
8.	Give or receive a patient handover to transition care responsibility.
9.	Collaborate as a member of an interprofessional team.
10.	Recognize a patient requiring urgent or emergent care and initiate evaluation and management.
11.	Obtain informed consent for tests and or procedure.
12.	Perform the general procedures of a physician.
13.	Identify system failures and contribute to a culture of safety and improvement.

Source: Association of American Medical Colleges, Selection from "Table of Contents," Core Entrustable Professional Activities for Entering Residency: Curriculum Developers' Guide, p. 1. Copyright © 2023 by Association of American Medical Colleges.

Medical education continues to evolve into a more robust and dynamic model. In 2017, the AAMC introduced the Emerging Areas in Medicine Competency Series, including Quality Improvement and Patient Safety Competencies (QIPS), Telehealth, and Diversity and Inclusion modules. In 2018, the Accreditation Council for Graduate Medical Education's (ACGMEs) Milestones 2.0 began. Its focus was on interpersonal and communications skills, problem-based learning and improvement, professionalism, and a systems-based practice approach.

In 2020, Action Plan 1 of the AAMC Strategic Plan was announced. This platform aims to strengthen medical education with a competency-based approach. However, it still has a long way to go in teaching effective communication skills such as motivational interviewing.

DOs follow a slightly different course of education. There is a long history of tension between MDs and DOs. Although osteopathic medicine was founded in the 1800s, it did not become acceptable until the mid-20th century. Up until the 1960s and 1970s most hospitals did not grant DOs hospital privileges, which greatly impacted their practice. By the 1980s these issues had been resolved, and most hospitals saw either profession as a viable option. One of the main differences between the two professions is the guiding principles of osteopathic medicine:

- They consider the entire body as a unit, which encompasses the mind, body, and spirit.
- They recognize the body can regulate itself and include self-healing properties and health maintenance.
- How we are built and how we function are interrelated.
- Treatment is based on an understanding of the body and how all these components are interrelated.

According to the American Academy of Credentialing for Osteopathic Medicine (AACOM), these principles are incorporated into the seven pillars of education that guide their curriculum, with only one of those pillars focused on interpersonal and communication skills: clear effective communication, shared decision-making, and cultural competency. The osteopathic model appears more holistic in approach than the MD pathway, as it takes into consideration the whole person including the mind, body, and spirit. Training appears to foster a deeper connection with patients and their families. However, communication and listening skills are still suboptimal; the focus is still more on providing advice, education, and counseling, considering the patient's wishes, and involving them in the decision-making process.

PAs receive medical education after completing a bachelor's degree. They have prerequisite requirements within the sciences before they can apply to the program, but the bachelor's degree can be in any profession. Their training follows the medical model, and after graduation they practice under the license of their supervising physician. A PA's education appears to be more robust when it comes to communication skills, which involve simulated experiences as well as hands-on learning. Within their core competencies, proficiency in interpersonal and communication skills is required. They must establish meaningful therapeutic relationships with patients and families to ensure patients' values and preferences are considered. They must communicate effectively as well as demonstrate sensitivity, honesty, and compassion in all conversations as well as understand the emotions, behaviors, and responses of others, which allow for effective interpersonal interactions. They also much recognize communication barriers and provide solutions, which is similar to the other two models, but what sets them apart is their module on education involving person-centered care, which includes eliciting and acknowledging the story of the individual and applying the context of the individuals life to their care, including environmental and cultural influences, as well as counseling, educating, and empowering patients and families to participate in their care and enable shared decision-making (National Commission on Certification of Physician Assistants [NCCPA] et al., 2021).

All three of these educational pathways (MD, DO, PA) consider effective communication and listening important but do not include education on what that truly is. They discuss shared decision-making as if the providers are still the ones responsible for the health care plan and the patients appear to be bystanders who give input. There is a big difference between *patient-centered care* and *patient-driven care,* which we will explore further in the chapters to come.

Table 2.3 **Communication Skills Comparison Chart**

	MD	DO	PA
Active listening	x	x	
Listening to understand	x		
Communicating effectively	x	x	x
Recognizing communication barriers	x		x
Counseling/educating	x	x	x
Demonstrating compassion	x	x	x
Demonstrating insight into human emotion	x		x
Using patient-centered language		x	
Understanding person-centered language			
Establishing meaningful therapeutic relationships with patients and families			x
Shared decision-making			x

Sources: AACOM (2024); AAMC (n.d.b.); Englander et al. (2013); NCCPA et al. (2021)

The Office Visit

In a typical office visit a consultation would look something like this: The provider will ask questions and gather data from the patient regarding their medical condition or chief complaint. They will do an examination and determine the best course of action, order any necessary tests and provide education and prescriptions to treat the condition that they are seeing. The patient may walk away from the encounter feeling less than cared for. A metanalysis from Ericksen et al. (2023) looked at patients' negative experiences from primary studies, which included 24 reports revealing four themes:

Theme 1: Problems With Access to Care

- Patients complained about not being able to get appointments.
- Patients complained of having a delay in diagnosis, which led to suffering, poorer health, and even death.
- Patients complained of continuity of care being suboptimal.

Theme 2: Failure to Get Information

- Patients found it difficult to get enough information about a specific diagnosis or treatment from the provider.
- Patients found the information given to them difficult to understand.
- Patients found they had no time to ask questions.
- Patients complained about receiving contradicting information from different providers.
- Patients found it difficult and awkward to ask questions.
- Patients were insecure about how they should act in the patient-provider relationship.

Theme 3: Inappropriate or Bad Treatment

- Patients felt providers lacked respect for them.
- Patients felt like they were being treated as a diagnosis rather than a person.
- Patients felt providers lacked empathy.
- Patients felt a lack of emotional support from providers.
- Patients felt health care professionals abused their power.
- Patients reported they had to fight to be believed.
- Patients reported doubting themselves because of how they were being treated.

Theme 4: Problem Trusting Health Care Providers

- Patients have lost trust in the medical system.
- Patients avoided health care services.
- Patients delayed treatment because of bad experiences.

- Patients felt helpless in a system of bureaucracy.
- Patients wanted justice.
- Patients wanted those responsible for injustice to admit wrongdoing.
- Patients did not want what happened to them to happen to others.

Let's go back to Lynette's encounter with the radiologist giving her mammogram results; you can see she had a lot of the same complaints that are listed in Eriksen's (2023) meta-analysis. She had to fight for the information she needed, she did not feel heard but dismissed and angry; she wanted the radiologist to see how they were treating her and making her feel; and she did not want this to happen to anyone else.

In the next chapter, we will look at a different model of care and learning. Nurses are trained in a very different way from the beginning of their journey.

KEY POINTS

- The medical model or expert model has its roots in a paternalistic model.
- Medical education core competencies focus mainly on scientific processes.
- Providers are the experts of medical information.
- Patients are the experts of their lives.

QUESTIONS FOR REFLECTION

- Galileo Galilei said, "We cannot teach people anything; we can only help them discover it within themselves." What does this mean to you?
- What type of provider do you see yourself as?
- What do you want your patients to say about their interactions with you?
- How will you show your patients that you care?
- What will be the core competencies of your practice?

SUGGESTED ACTIVITIES

1. Role-play scenarios. Have students explore both good and bad health care experiences and role-play them in front of the class. Ask the class to discuss what was different in each scenario. Which provider would they want to see and why?
2. Group discussion and debates
    a. Who is responsible for the

outcomes of health, the patient or the provider?
   b. What part do insurance companies play in making providers feel like they are responsible?
   c. How do patient surveys impact providers?
3. Case study analysis. Provide participants with a case study highlighting both the paternalist and patient-centered model. Have students work in groups to analyze the case, the outcomes, cost savings, and patient engagement and make recommendations based on their analysis.
4. Reflective journals. Have students discuss, with different providers (e.g., MD, DO, PA), what their feelings are about patients who do not follow recommendations. How do they handle these situations? What is similar or different about their approach? Have them discuss what is important to them about patient outcomes.

References

Association of American Medical Colleges. (n.d.a.). *Core EPA publications and presentations*. https://www.aamc.org/what-we-do/mission-areas/medical-education/cbme/core-epas/publications

Association of American Medical Colleges. (n.d.b.). *The premed competencies and what they mean*. https://students-residents.aamc.org/media/15396/download

Association of American Medical Colleges, American Association of Colleges of Osteopathic Medicine, & Accreditation Council for Graduate Medical Education. (2024). *Foundational competencies for undergraduate medical education*. https://image.email.aamc.org/lib/fe8e13727c63047f73/m/1/3d55a3aa-b3ba-4c14-a447-8c60e27a6f05.pdf

Berger, B. A., & Villaume, W. A. (2020). Why another book on motivational interviewing? In *Motivational interviewing for health care professionals: A sensible approach* (2nd ed.pp. 1–9). American Pharmacists Association. https://doi.org/10.21019/9781582123219

Cliff, B. (2012). The evolution of patient-centered care. *Journal of Healthcare Management*, *57*(2), 86–88.

Cushing, A. (1999). Origin of the medical model. *Collegian*, *6*(1), i. https://doi.org/10.1016/s1322-7696(08)60317-0

Englander, R., Cameron, T., Ballard, A. J., Dodge, J., Bull, J., & Aschenbrener, C. A. (2013). Toward a common taxonomy of competency domains for the health professions and competencies for physicians. *Academic Medicine*, *88*(8), 1088–1094. https://doi.org/10.1097/acm.0b013e31829a3b2b

Eriksen, A., Fegran, L., Fredwall, T., & Larsen, I. (2023). Patients' negative experiences with health care settings brought to light by formal complaints: A qualitative metasynthesis. *Journal of Clinical Nursing*, *32*(17–18), 5816–5835. https://doi.org/10.1111/jocn.16704

Narsaria, R. (2015, March 10). *The Hippocratic oath: The original and revised version*. The Practo Blog for Doctors. https://doctors.practo.com/the-hippocratic-oath-the-original-and-revised-version/

National Commission on Certification of Physician Assistants, Accreditation Review Commission on Education for the Physician Assistant, American Academy of PAs, & Physician Assistant Education Association. (2021). *Competencies for the PA profession*. https://www.aapa.org/download/90503/

Chapter 3

The Collaborative Approach to Patient Care

Caring is the essence of nursing.

—Jean Watson

This chapter will introduce readers to the world of collaborative patient care through a nursing education lens. It will illustrate why working collaboratively with your patient is most effective. We will also explore how this version of collaboration may look different than other versions. We will look at concepts we have to let go of as providers that may be held closely in the nursing model and how we need to let the patient lead.

OBJECTIVES

- Students will be able to connect the nursing process to patient-centered care.
- Students will be able to understand the differences between RN and APRN education.
- Students will be able to explain the transition from being an RN to entering APRN practice.
- Students will explore evidence-based communication strategies.
- Students will begin to explore patient-centered care in a different way, helping patients become more engaged in lifestyle changes.
- Students will become familiar with the term "compassionomics" and be able to give some examples of how utilizing compassion in health care has positive benefits both for the patient and the provider.

KEY TERMS AND DEFINITIONS

- **Nursing process:** A systematic, patient-centered approach in nursing that involves five steps: assessment, diagnosis (problems), outcome planning, implementation, and evaluation. It focuses of the nursing process is to understand the patient holistically, including physical, psychological, sociocultural, spiritual, economic, and lifestyle factors.
- **Maslow's hierarchy of needs:** Maslow's hierarchy of needs is a psychological framework that prioritizes human needs, starting with basic physiological needs (e.g., food, water, sleep) and progressing to higher-level needs like self-esteem and self-actualization. This model is used in the nursing process to prioritize care.
- **Clinical judgment model:** A revised model of the nursing process that places more emphasis on critical thinking and decision-making skills. It includes six steps: recognizing cues, analyzing cues, prioritizing hypotheses, generating solutions, acting, and evaluating outcomes.
- **Next-Generation NCLEX (NGN):** The NCLEX is a national exam for registered nurses that they must pass before becoming licensed and incorporates the clinical judgment model to assess critical thinking and decision-making skills.
- **Advanced practice nursing (APRN):** Nursing with extended medical education, allowing them to practice at a higher level of care. Focus is still holistic care but includes diagnosis and management of disease states, much like a provider.
- **American Association of Colleges of Nursing (AACN) Essentials:** The AACN is a credentialing body that has developed a set of core competencies for nursing education, including domains like person-centered care, quality and safety, professionalism, and interprofessional partnerships.
- **Value-based reimbursement model:** A repayment system for providers that is based and incentivized by patient outcomes and quality metrices such as improved diabetic or hypertensive control or a reduction in obesity.
- **Compassionomics:** A term developed by Dr. Stephen Trzeciak and Dr. Anthony Mazzarelli who pioneered and systematically studied the measurable effects of compassionate care in a health care setting.

Educating the RN: The Nursing Process

The **nursing process** has always involved patient-centered care. From the beginning of nursing school, starting at the undergraduate level, nurses are taught about how the body works and how to prevent disease and engage people in the healing process. Fundamental to the nursing process is caring about the patient, including displaying mutual respect and developing a trusting relationship, which includes a robust education around effective communication.

Nurses are taught that communication skills are both verbal and nonverbal, including culture and spiritual aspects in the bachelorette program. Nurses utilize the nursing process to help teach patients and learn from them. Specifically, the nursing process involves the following five steps: assessment, diagnosis (problems), outcome planning, implementation, and evaluation. Assessment is the first tool that a nurse is trained to do. This includes the physical aspects of the person and considers everything about the person, including "psychological, sociocultural, spiritual, economic, and lifestyle factors," which may impact patients' health (American Nurses Association [ANA], 2017). Diagnoses, later changed to analysis, are based on the nurse's clinical judgment regarding problems that they see could arise. It guides the patient's nursing care plan. For example, let's look at an elderly patient who is bedridden because of pneumonia.

- Assessment: Skin integrity
- Diagnosis (problem): Potential for skin breakdown
- Outcome planning: Patient will remain free from skin breakdown
- Implementation: Turn patient every 2 hours
- Evaluation: Patient skin is free from skin breakdown (ANA, 2017)

Nursing diagnoses were first introduced in the 1950s and involved clinical judgment about a problem, which differed from a medical diagnosis, which is about a condition or disease. It gave nurses a common language to work with. A complete list can be found at nandadiagnoses.com. However, using the term "diagnosis" was confusing; the more common term used today is "nursing problems." Many of these nursing problems are based on **Maslow's hierarchy of needs**. Abraham Maslow was an American psychologist who is considered a founding father of humanistic psychology and is best known for his theory of motivation based on a hierarchy of needs. He proposed that we must first satisfy basic needs before we are motivated to fulfill higher needs. For example, if someone is worried about where they will sleep that night or where their next meal is coming from, they might not be as concerned about their purpose in life or the legacy they will leave. In nursing, this framework helps us prioritize patients' care plans. More about Maslow will be discussed in Chapter 5.

Basic Physiological Needs

Example: Imbalanced nutrition—less than body requirements

- Food: Evaluate their nutritional status. Find out what they like, what they don't like.
- Water: Evaluate hydration status. Find out preferred drinks or beverages.
- Toileting: Make sure toileting needs are met.

- Breathing: Maintain an adequate airway and provide comfort.
- Circulation: Maintain adequate circulation.
- Sleep: Provide an environment conducive to sleep.
- Exercise: Evaluate exercise needs; find out preferences.

Safety and Security

Example: Risk for falls

- Injury prevention: Make sure call light within reach, pathway is clear, home is safe.
- Fostering a climate of trust and safety: Listen to your patient, keep information confidential, and provide privacy.
- Patient education: When asked, provide education on subjects that may be unclear to patients.

Love and Belonging

Example: Anxiety

- Fostering supportive relationships: Provide comfort, understanding, empathy.
- Avoiding social isolation: Be present for the patient. Ask about their social networks and support systems.
- Listening to understand: Try to understand the patient and what they need.
- Therapeutic communication techniques: Communicate empathy, warmth, understanding, and nonjudgment to your patient. Invite them into discussions about what strengths they possess, what coping skills work for them, and what strategies might be best for them moving forward.

Self-Esteem

Example: Situational low self-esteem

- Acceptance: Demonstrate acceptance and nonjudgment of your patient. Encourage patients to work toward acceptance of self.
- Offer positive reinforcement for any strengths that you see within the patient.
- Build up and draw out their ideas to work toward solutions.

Self-Actualization

Example: Readiness for enhanced hope

- Empowerment: Work toward empowering patients to master their circumstances.

- Reaching maximum potential: Encourage lifelong growth and learning.

As you can see from this model, nurses are trained from the beginning to use clinical judgment as it applies to the whole patient and consider all the problems that could arise and have a plan to address them, which includes considering what the patient needs and wants, making the training process for nurses much more patient centered from the beginning of the program.

Clinical Judgment Model

Today, the nursing process model has been revised to a **clinical judgment model**, which is reflected in the **Next-Generation NCLEX (NGN)** national exam that all nurses must pass at the end of their bachelorette training to become a registered nurse (RN). This new model motivates nursing schools across America to develop curriculum in ways nurses can be more prepared to do critical analysis and become competent in their clinical judgment. This change was brought on from the realization that graduate nurses still missed many important clues, even though they passed the national certification exam, which put patients in jeopardy.

To address the deficit in critical analysis we turn to Patricia Benner's research in 1983, with her introduction of the *Novice to Expert Model*. Her research demonstrated that nurses moved from being a novice to an expert in a predictable pattern. The more experience a nurse gained, the easier it became for them to recognize cues and put them together, allowing them to react to a situation, utilizing their experience and ultimately increasing their competence.

Chris Tanner's work added to this by introducing the clinical judgment model in 2004, which demonstrated a four-step process involved in nursing judgement including noticing a problem, interpreting what this means, responding appropriately, and evaluating the outcome. Ultimately, the following six-step process is known officially as the National Council of State Board of Nursing (NCSBN) clinical judgment measurement model (NCJMM).

1. Recognize the cues: Can you see what is happening and recognize it?
2. Analyze cues: Do you know what they mean?
3. Prioritize hypotheses: Can you order what you think is happening?
4. Generate solutions: Can you figure out the next steps?
5. Take action: Can you prioritize the most important things to do first?
6. Evaluate outcomes: Can you reflect on what happened and see how it is related to what you did?

Communication Skills

Through nursing education, nursing students learn about communicating with their patients in a therapeutic way, both in the classroom and in clinical practice when they are with patients. They are taught to be their patients' advocates and learn the essential skills that are involved in a therapeutic relationship. Once they have graduated, they continue to grow and learn at the bedside. They understand the disease process; they give medications and watch their effects. They have explained to the patients and their families what the provider said and what it means. They have held the hands of their patients and loved ones at some of the most heart-wrenching times, expressing empathy and compassion. They have also served as mentors to their patients, teaching them about their disease process, medications, and follow-up care, and have learned to interact in effective ways to help patients become their healthiest selves. Many of them have practiced at the bedside for years before entering an advanced practice program. Patient-centered care is at the very core of their practice.

Education for Advanced Practice Registered Nursing

As a nurse begins advanced practice training, which includes another 2 to 3 years of study, gaining a master's degree, they enter a provider role. This is a new world for them. They add to the years of training they received as undergraduates learning now how to incorporate the diagnosing and treatment of disease. This includes learning the medical model and thinking like a provider. In April 2021, the American Association of Colleges of Nursing (AACN) published *The Essentials: Core Competencies for Professional Nursing Education*. These changes came about from recent studies that showed that registered and advanced practice nurses were less prepared for the rigors of the job. The document is 82 pages long and includes the following 10 domains:

1. Knowledge for nursing practice
2. Person-centered care
3. Population health
4. Scholarship for nursing discipline
5. Quality and safety
6. Interprofessional partnerships
7. Systems-based practice
8. Informatics and healthcare technologies
9. Professionalism
10. Personal, professional, and leadership development

Looking specifically at domain 2, person-centered care, let's compare the essential components at both the bachelorette and master's degree level (Table 3.1; AACN, 2023).

Table 3.1 **American Academy Nursing Credentialing Essentials in Education**

Entry-Level Professional Nursing Education	Advanced-Level Nursing Education
2.1. Engage with the individual in establishing a caring relationship	
2.1a. Demonstrate qualities of empathy	2.1d. Promote caring relationships to effect positive outcomes
2.1b. Demonstrate compassionate care	2.1e. Foster caring relationships
2.1c. Establish mutual respect with the individual and family	
2.2. Communicate effectively with individuals	
2.2a. Demonstrate relationship-centered care	2.2g. Demonstrate advanced communication skills and techniques using a variety of modalities with diverse audiences
2.2b. Consider individual beliefs, values, and personalized information in communications	2.2h. Design evidence-based, person-centered engagement materials
2.2c. Use a variety of communication modes appropriate for the context	2.2i. Apply individualized information, such as genetic/genomic, pharmacogenetic, and environmental exposure information in the delivery of personalized health care
2.2d. Demonstrate the ability to conduct sensitive or difficult conversations	2.2j. Facilitate difficult conversations and disclosure of sensitive information
2.2e. Use evidence-based patient teaching materials, considering health literacy, vision, hearing, and cultural sensitivity	
2.2ff. Demonstrate emotional intelligence in communications	

Entry-Level Professional Nursing Education	**Advanced-Level Nursing Education**
2.3. Integrate assessment skills in practice	
2.3a. Create an environment during assessment that promotes a dynamic interactive experience	2.3h. Demonstrate that one's practice is informed by a comprehensive assessment appropriate to the functional area of advanced nursing practice
2.3b. Obtain a complete and accurate history in a systematic manner	
2.3c. Perform a clinically relevant, holistic health assessment	
2.3d. Perform point of care screening/diagnostic testing (e.g., blood glucose, P02, EKG)	
2.3e. Distinguish between normal and abnormal health findings	
2.3f. Apply nursing knowledge to gain a holistic perspective of the person, family, community, and population	
2.3g. Communicate findings of a comprehensive assessment	
2.4. Diagnose actual or potential health problems and needs	
2.4a. Synthesize assessment data in the context of the individual's current preferences, situation, and experience	2.4f. Employ context-driven, advanced reasoning to the diagnostic and decision-making process
2.4b. Create a list of problems/health concerns	2.4g. Integrate advanced scientific knowledge to guide decision-making

Entry-Level Professional Nursing Education	**Advanced-Level Nursing Education**
2.4c. Prioritize problems / health concerns	
2.4d. Understand and apply the results of social screening, psychological testing, laboratory data, imaging studies, and other diagnostic tests in actions and plans of care	
2.4e. Contribute as a team member to the formation and improvement of diagnoses	
2.5. Develop a plan of care	
2.5a. Engage the individual and the team in plan development	2.5h. Lead and collaborate with an interprofessional team to develop a comprehensive plan of care
2.5b. Organize care based on mutual health goals	2.5i. Prioritize risk mitigation strategies to prevent or reduce adverse outcomes
2.5c. Prioritize care based on best evidence	2.5j. Develop evidence-based interventions to improve outcomes and safety
2.5d. Incorporate evidence-based interventions to improve outcomes and safety	2.5k. Incorporate innovations into practice when evidence is not available
2.5e. Anticipate outcomes of care (expected, unexpected, and potentially adverse)	
2.5f. Demonstrate rationale for plan	
2.5g. Address individuals' experiences and perspectives in designing plans of care	

Entry-Level Professional Nursing Education	**Advanced-Level Nursing Education**
2.6 Demonstrate accountability for care delivery	
2.6a. Implement individual plan of care using established protocols	2.6e. Model best care practices to the team
2.6b. Communicate care delivery though multiple modalities	2.6f. Monitor aggregate metrics to assure accountability for care outcomes
2.6c. Delegate appropriately to team members	2.6g. Promote delivery of care that supports practice at the full scope of education
2.6d. Monitor the implementation of the plan of care.	2.6h. Contribute to the development of policies and processes that promote transparency and accountability
	2.6i. Apply current and emerging evidence to the development of care guidelines/tools
	2.6j. Ensure accountability throughout transitions of care across the health continuum
2.7. Evaluate outcomes of care	
2.7a. Reassess the individual to evaluate health outcomes/goals	2.7d. Analyze data to identify gaps and inequities in care and monitor trends in outcomes
2.7b. Modify plan of care as needed	2.7e. Monitor epidemiological and system-level aggregate data to determine health care outcomes and trends
2.7c. Recognize the need for modifications to standard practice	2.7f. Synthesize outcome data to inform evidence-based practice, guidelines, and policies

Entry-Level Professional Nursing Education	Advanced-Level Nursing Education
2.8. Promote self-care management	
2.8a. Assist the individual to engage in self-care management	2.8f. Develop strategies that promote self-care management
2.8b. Employ individualized educational strategies based on learning theories, methodologies, and health literacy	2.8g. Incorporate the use of current and emerging technologies to support self-care management
2.8c. Educate individuals and families regarding self-care for health promotion, illness prevention, and illness management	2.8h. Employ counseling techniques, including motivational interviewing, to advance wellness and self-care management
2.8d. Respect individuals and families' self-determination in their health care decisions	2.8i. Evaluate adequacy of resources available to support self-care management
2.8e. Identify personal, system, and community resources available to support self-care management	2.8j. Foster partnerships with community organizations to support self-care management
2.9. Provide care coordination	
2.9a. Facilitate continuity of care based on assessment of assets and needs	2.9f. Evaluate communication pathways among providers and others across settings, systems, and communities
2.9b. Communicate with relevant stakeholders across health systems	2.9g. Develop strategies to optimize care coordination and transitions of care
2.9c. Promote collaboration by clarifying responsibilities among individual, family, and team members	2.9h. Guide the coordination of care across health systems
2.9d. Recognize when additional expertise and knowledge is needed to manage the patient	2.9i. Analyze system-level and public policy influence on care coordination

Entry-Level Professional Nursing Education	Advanced-Level Nursing Education
2.9e. Provide coordination of care of individuals and families in collaboration with care team.	2.9j. Participate in system-level changes to improve care coordination across settings

Source: American Association of Colleges of Nursing, "Domain 2: Person-Centered Care," The Essentials: Core Competencies for Professional Nursing Education, pp. 29–32. Copyright © 2021 by American Association of Colleges of Nursing (AACN). Reprinted with permission.

For both RN and APRN education, you can see the emphasis placed on developing a relationship with the patient and utilizing effective communication skills, to include motivational interviewing in the APRN tract. Nurses are taught these things at the undergraduate level. They have 600 clinical hours to practice these skills before becoming an RN; then they must practice between 1 and 2 years *before* they can go further into the APRN tract of education, giving them a robust education in how to interact with patients and their families.

The Transition

The process of transitioning from a nurse to advanced practice is well studied and can be an anxiety-producing time. Nurses step out of their expert role and find themselves lost in a sea of knowledge that can be daunting. First-year nurse practitioner (NP) students are what I like to term the "deer in the headlight" cohort. The saying "you don't know what you don't know" really applies here. Up until this point every patient a nurse has interacted with has had a medical diagnosis by a provider. Now the responsibility of that medical diagnosis is up to the NP, and with only symptoms to go on, multiple diagnoses are possible.

An activity I often use with my nursing students to illustrate this principle begins with a patient scenario with the complaints of itchy watery eyes. These symptoms are classic textbook allergic conjunctivitis. In working up the patient, the students can go down multiple pathways to diagnosing it correctly, all the way to an emergent eye condition. It is the perfect example to introduce them to the world of diagnosing because, based just on symptoms, diagnosing can be overwhelming, and they begin to *see* all that they do not know.

Provider Responsibilities

Taking on the responsibilities of a provider can feel overwhelming, and some students will not be able to effectively make this transition. Instead, they will revert to the nursing role they feel expert in. But those who persist will find that their nursing education and skills are still very applicable; they just need to shift their focus.

One thing I like to tell nurses in that "deer in the headlight semester" is the following: "In the MD, DO, and PA tract they have not touched a patient before year 5 of their education. They do not know medical terms, drugs, physical assessment or how to interview or talk to a patient or family. Then, in medical school they learn all of it in that short time. Residency is when they get better at it. As nurses you have had all that background training, and you have utilized it. You know how to talk to patients and families, how to examine them, how to give medications and what those medications do. What you are lacking is how to diagnose and treat illness, so don't forget to bring your nursing skills with you as you enter this role. You will be surprised at how fast you will pick things up and how quickly your library of cases will fill up, so you will be able to pull from that experience to guide you." This pep talk seems to help, and by the time they are at the end of their training you can see the transition as they begin to gain some confidence.

The transition process involves learning how to *think* like a provider. **Advanced practice nursing** students must learn the medical model of documenting, billing, and systematically developing diagnosis with plans of care, all of which are billable activities, something as nurses they did not have to consider. They are counseled that at each visit they need to discuss obesity and tobacco cessation with the appropriate billing codes because you get paid extra for it. Payment to providers and hospitals is also influenced by results. For example, every year the Centers for Medicare & Medicaid Services can penalize hospitals that have high readmission rates. In 2023, 60% of U.S. hospitals received a financial penalty. This penalty was the result of the Affordable Care Act of 2010 (Allen, 2023). (If you want to know how your hospital is faring, you can look up your hospital in your state by going to kffhealthnews.org/news/hospital-penalties/.)

The thought behind this is if the patients with high-risk conditions for readmission are treated properly, they will not be admitted within 30 days for the same condition, which could be partly true but not wholly. In fact, most readmission is because of noncompliance. For example, let's look at a condition that causes common readmission, such as congestive heart failure or diabetes. Both conditions require specific medications to be taken at a given time as well as following a specific diet. Success depends on the patient following those instructions. We know this because when in the hospital on a controlled, specified diet and taking the right medications on time their conditions improve, but when they go home they get out of control again. Lifestyle changes are hard. People are accustomed to eating a certain way and drinking a certain drink, and many forget to take their medications as prescribed, especially as they age. Hospitals have invested heavily in ways to prevent readmission rates from these high-risk diseases to ensure patient success, but as we've learned, engaging patients in follow-through is key. We can control certain things in the hospital, but how can we help them implement strategies that will work for them once they are at home?

Let's look at this system in private practice. Under the **value-based reimbursement model** providers are evaluated by different quality metrics such as hemoglobin A1c levels for their diabetic patients, BMI in their obese patients, blood pressure for patients who have diagnosis of high blood pressure, and so on. There is an incentive for providers to improve these metrics with a pay-for-performance contract, which gives bonuses or increased reimbursements for better outcomes. The problem with these models is they place the ownership of the problem with the providers. That is not where the problem lies. With this model we now have an atmosphere that is provider centered rather than patient centered. According to Berger and Villaume (2019) there are multiple themes a provider thinks about when they have this type of relationship with their patients:

- "I just need to tell my patients what to do."
- "I just need to educate my patients."
- "It is my job to motivate my patients."
- "I need to empower my patients."
- "I need to fix or save my patients."
- "I do disease management."
- "My patients lie to me."
- "I feel like I'm wrestling with my patients."
- "I am the expert here."
- "My patients are difficult and often in denial."

Unfortunately, disease management is not as simple as just educating someone or telling them what to do or giving them the pep talk. The results from this type of communication on lifestyle changes are usually less than desirable, with unhappy patients who do not feel heard or empowered and frustrated providers who are continually met with suboptimal results and feel as if they are in some kind of power struggle with their patients, and it is *not* what they went into medicine for.

National studies have shown that up to 50% of providers feel burned out, with outpatient providers feeling more emotionally exhausted (Martinez-Hollingsworth et al., 2023). Once a provider can shift their mindset from the goal of patient compliance to getting to know their patients better and helping them make better decisions for their own care, great things can happen. Patient satisfaction scores will improve *and* patient compliance will increase (Shute, 2019).

Building a Relationship

As a provider, you will see your patients over an extended time. Even in the hospital setting you can have repeat admissions that allow you to get to know a patient and their family. Building a relationship takes time, but the first step in this relationship involves getting to know your patient's story. Focus on the person in front of you more than the disease they are coming in for. Get to know them, their family, and their personal struggles. If you genuinely care about the person, it will come through and they will feel it. When you listen, try to see things from their point of view, not from your point of view. While working in rural health I saw many things and had opportunities to build such relationships. One of my patients who had been bitten by a dog showed up on a tractor. It was freezing outside, and after we bandaged him up my nurse drove him home, so he did not try to go home on his tractor and freeze to death.

One of the most memorable experiences I had in rural health was with a patient who came into our clinic who had cut his thumb badly opening a can. He was on a blood thinner, so he was bleeding a lot. Normally, I would bandage him up and send him to the ER, which was about 15 miles down the road, but he was bleeding too severely. I had to stitch him up. I knew how to put in stitches, but it had been a long time since I had done it, so my memory was not as good as it once was. Between me and my nurse we managed to do a pretty good job, bandaged him up, and sent him on his way. As I was reviewing the steps in my mind after he left, I realized that I did not put a nonstick dressing over his stitches, which would probably cause the stitches to stick over the weekend. My nurse and I talked about it, and since we were slow that day, we decided to pack up a bag of supplies and redress his wound at the Fish Fry. He was busily cooking up the fish as we walked in and was surprised to see us. We asked if he would mind if we redressed his thumb. He complied, and we were on our way. We felt better about a job well done, and he was grateful knowing how much we cared about him—enough so that we would close office, pack up a bag, and find him so we could make things right.

Each patient is unique and has a special story. We as providers are privileged to be part of some of the most special and hard times of their lives. I made it a point to listen to each patient and help in every way I could. If I had bad news for a patient, I took the time to have them come in so that we could talk, and I had the time to answer all their questions. More than one time I had the results of their tests, which showed a cancer was growing, and these visits were hard to get through because I knew them and I cared. If I knew someone was waiting on test results and I got them, they would get a call from me telling them how things were. We were in this journey together.

I have carried this practice into the hospitals where you don't get to see patients repeatedly to build a relationship, but I have found if I listen and try to understand what it is they want or need and then ask permission to share knowledge or stories with them to help them understand better it is much better received and they are grateful. Patients want to feel heard and cared for. Having compassion for our patients and serving them has untold benefits not only for them, but evidence shows that there are benefits for us as well.

Compassion Matters

Dr. Stephen Trzechiak and Dr Anthony Mazzarelli have provided an abundance of evidence-based practice that shows the benefits to patients and providers in utilizing the simple tool of compassion with far-reaching effects—so much so that it can be life changing. ***Compassiononics*** is a book that highlights the results of their long study and was published in 2019 by the Studer Group. Dr. Trzechiak has gone on to speak at multiple organizations and conference events highlighting their findings. I had the pleasure of being at one of them.

According to Tzzechiak and Mazzerelli (2019), it all began when Dr. Mazzarelli was tasked as the new chief executive officer (CEO) at Cooper University Hospital to improve patient satisfaction scores. Improved satisfaction scores would increase the bottom line for the hospital from reimbursement rates and improve their ratings. As any good CEO does, he called in a focus group to see if they could identify the problem that was causing low patient satisfaction scores. The recommendations were not surprising and came back with suggestions, including having providers be more compassionate toward patients. Realizing this was going to be a hard sell to the providers who would feel they were doing the best they could, he solicited the help of his long-time colleague and friend Dr. Trzechiak, an intensivist who was actively involved in research. His thought was if Dr. Trzechiak could find evidence that compassion mattered in measurable ways it might be more convincing to providers and be the vehicle that could invoke change.

At first, Dr. Trzechiak was not enthused with this research endeavor as the problem is not a new one and not easy to solve; however, his interest was sparked later that week when his son was working on a project from school and asked for his help. The project involved his son doing a presentation on what he felt was the most pressing problem of our time. This question got Trzechiak thinking and asking himself if he was working on the *most* important problem of our time with his research.

Ultimately, Trzechiak decided to take up the research to show that providing health care with compassion was beneficial and had measurable results. He did not think it would take very long, but in the end took several years as he plodded his way through the mountain of research on the subject. In the end, the research design involved a qualitative systematic review with "reference of references" methodology, including 1,000 scientific abstracts and 250 research papers. Key scientific studies were captured, including from Harvard Medical School and the *New England Journal of Medicine*, and the results showed a wave of evidence that could not be denied. Compassion matters not only in positive measurable ways to patient outcomes, but surprisingly there are health benefits to the provider as well, including less provider burnout.

With this evidence, the trajectory of Dr. Trezechiak's life changed, for at that moment he knew what the most important problem of our time was, and he devoted his life to help change it. What he found was we are in a compassion crisis. To illustrate this point, here are some of the things he found:

- Meta-analysis with 13,000 undergraduate studies shows lack of empathy is increasing among students.

- A Harvard University survey showed out of 10,000 U.S. middle and high school students, nearly two thirds of the youth said their parents valued achievements and accolades over caring about them.
- A Pew research study showed one third of all Americans do not consider compassion to be a core value.
- One half of Americans do not consider U.S. health care and providers compassionate.
- Sixty-three percent of health care providers say they have observed a decline in compassion over the past 5 years.
- Sixty-four percent of U.S patients said they have had a patient encounter that lacked compassion—with similar data in Ireland and the UK (Trzeciak & Mazzarelli, 2019).

Empathy versus Compassion

There is a difference between being empathetic and being compassionate. According to Trzeciak and Mazzarelli (2019), "compassion" is an action word involving authentic caring, whereas "empathy" involves feeling what another is going through without necessarily doing anything about it. Developing a relationship with our patient's authenticity is paramount. A patient can tell if you truly care about them or are just putting up a façade. Caring is not something you can fake. It is something that is felt.

What did the evidence show? Here is a list of some of the physical benefits of utilizing a compassionate approach found in the studies reviewed by Trzeciak and Mazzarelli (2019):

- Compassion tripled the chance of recovery from heart attack.
- Compassion improved recovery from illness.
- Compassion improved surgical outcomes.
- Compassion decreased the pain response and need for pain medication.
- Compassion decreased the cortisol response, which decreased inflammation overall, improving long-term health consequences.
- Compassion lowered blood pressure.
- Compassion improved recovery from trauma.
- Compassion reduced back pain.
- Compassion reduced headaches.
- Compassion reduced irritable bowel syndrome.
- Patients who had providers who showed compassion had a 41% lower chance of serious complications from diabetes.

And these are just a partial list of the findings.

There were also psychological benefits in utilizing a compassionate approach:

- Compassion improved depression.

- Compassion improved anxiety.
- Compassion improved PTSD symptoms.
- Compassion made unbearable things more bearable (Trzeciak & Mazzarelli, 2019).

Based on the evidence, there are undeniable positive results shown for patients when a compassionate approach is utilized. But the benefits do not end with the patients. The surprising finding was how much benefit providers had from using a compassionate approach. Functional magnetic resonance imaging (fMRI) scans were done on providers to compare the effects on the brain when empathy was shown as opposed to compassion. Remember the difference between the two is feeling the patients pain versus being actively engaged in helping them. The empathetic approach lit up the pain center in the brain, meaning that when we are empathetic to someone, we will experience less pain ourselves, but the compassionate approach lit up the reward center of our brain. It's a dopamine hit for us!

Trzeciak and Mazzarelli (2023) wrote another book titled *Wonder Drug: 7 Scientifically Proven Ways That Serving Others Is the Best Medicine for Yourself.* We all know what dopamine does for us. It is our joy center, where time stops, where we want to be. Service can be very addictive to people. People who display higher levels of compassion in their job experience less burnout and more purpose. I have found this to be true in my own practice. I have found those of us who are more invested, more compassionate, see their job as a "calling" more than a job. Providers with this mentality did not feel the burnout of their counterparts. A "live to give" mentality scientifically improves all aspects of a person's life according to the evidence (Trzeciak & Mazzarelli, 2023).

Given the benefits of a compassionate approach to both the patient and the provider, why is it not an easy sell? Why do providers resist learning more about it? The answer lies in the fact that there is abundant data to show providers resist the idea that they are not compassionate for the following reasons:

- "I don't see it."
- "I don't have time."
- "I don't care."
- "I don't know how."
- "I don't believe it really matters." (Trzeciak & Mazzarelli, 2019, pp. 24–25)

Compassion Education

Multiple studies have shown that compassion can be taught *and* can be effective with just 40 seconds of an intervention (Bylund & Makoul, 2005; Dempsey, 2017; Fogarty et al., 1999; Roter et al., 1995). In a Johns Hopkins University study involving oncology patients, a randomized clinical trial was done with patients randomized to an oncologist utilizing the standard approach versus an appointment with an oncologist who added a compassionate statement at the beginning of the encounter and the end of the encounter. The measurement tool was a well-validated anxiety scale to see which approach produced less anxiety in the patient. The compassionate statement with the oncology patient included the following at the beginning: "I know this is a tough experience to go through and I want you to know that I am here with you. Some of the things that I say to you today may be difficult to understand, so I want you to feel comfortable in stopping me if something I say is confusing or doesn't make sense. We are here together, and we will go through this together." At the conclusion of the visit, the oncologist said, "I know this is a tough time for you and I want to emphasize again that we are in this together. I will be with you each step of the way" (Trzeciak & Mazzarelli, 2019, p. 251). The time it took for this intervention was roughly 40 seconds. Results from the compassionate interventional statement group showed patients felt more comfortable with the oncologist who used the compassionate statements and experienced less anxiety.

Think about the difference 40 seconds made in those patients' lives. Ask yourselves if you would be willing to invest 40 seconds of your time to help a patient in this way. More studies have shown that these brief interactions with compassionate statements can make a world of difference and dispel the myth that providers have used for years about not having enough time, when the research shows that 60%–90% of the time providers miss opportunities to be compassionate. When a patient says they are having a tough time, for example the provider does not dig deeper; in most cases they go on to the next problem (Trzeciak & Mazzarelli, 2019). Maybe the reason for this is their lack of comfort in this area or training, but the real question is "Can we afford not to get the training we need to be effective with compassionate statements in our practice?" More training in this area will benefit not only our patients but, as the evidence shows, providers as well.

Strengthening the Relationship

Once providers have established a relationship with a patient, it is important to nourish it. Again, being genuine and authentic is important. The following mixed-method study involved a systematic literature review of 73 studies and qualitative research activities, which found five practices that were found to enhance the relationship between the provider and the patient (Zulman et al., 2020):

- Providers need to take a moment prior to entering the room to prepare for the encounter. Review the last visit or the chart and then clear their mind and prepare to greet the patient. Do not appear hurried or rushed. It is helpful to put in notes that make a comment about something personal with the patient or family so that on the next visit they can ask the patient about it. For example, if the patient is going on vacation, starting school, getting married, or any other life event, make a comment in the note so that on review it will trigger the memory.

- Providers need to listen to understand not listen to reply. This includes sitting down, looking at the patient not the computer, leaning forward, and becoming engaged with their story. Let them teach you about who they are.
- Providers need to find out what matters most to the patient and not proceed with their own agenda.
- Providers need to connect to their patient's story and the backstory.
- Providers need to look for the emotional cues the patient is giving and notice them, name them, and validate the patients' emotions. Sometimes things are just hard, and we need to acknowledge that (Zulman et al., 2020).

This study reinforces many of the things you will learn through motivational interviewing and validates its value.

Patient-Driven Care: A New Model

Patients have more information and informational technology at their fingertips than ever before. Couple this with artificial intelligence and they are positioned to be in a place when true collaboration can take place, and they can be empowered to make changes in their lives. A new model of healthcare is emerging that puts the patient front and center, patient-driven care. Swan (2009) talks about three types of patient-driven care that are emerging. Figure 3.1 depicts how an individual (self) interacts within a multiple party system. Patients become the focus and can take ownership of various tasks of their health care, including tracking various variables such as blood pressure, weight, and hemoglobin a1c, and be active participants in researching their problems and coming up with solutions that work for them, with the help of their providers' expertise (Swan, 2009). This model represents the very essence of patient-driven care.

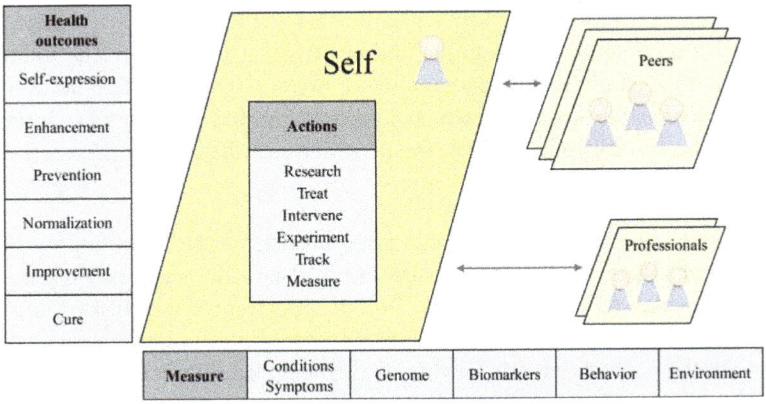

Figure 3.1 A new model of healthcare.

This model is exemplified in an experience my son Joe had with his health care provider. Joe often complained about going to see the doctor. He found the visits condescending and not worth his time. He did not see value in them, complaining often that he would not even know how much the visit was going to cost him until the bills arrived. These negative experiences kept him from seeking health care for years, but as technology has become more available and I being an NP he was able to educate himself and prepare for his doctor's visits more thoroughly in recent years. Now his visits are more patient driven. He goes in after he has thoroughly researched the subject on the internet with what he thinks is wrong given his symptoms, and then he calls me and discusses his ideas. I give him feedback he considers reliable, and then he goes to his provider. Now his provider treats him like a colleague more than a patient and listens to him, offering suggestions if she has another point she would like to make or wants to educate him on some facts that he may not have considered, and he listens to her. Now when he leaves he feels empowered, in control, and armed with increased knowledge, which he can then transform into a plan of action that will work for him. He now goes to the doctor more often. I believe we are now transitioning from patient-centered care to patient-driven care, which will be ultimately a much better and more successful model.

KEY POINTS

- Nurses are trained from day 1 to get to know their patients personally.
- Nursing educational essential competencies at both the bachelor's and master's level show extensive training in communications.
- APRN educational competencies are the only competencies that include motivational interviewing as a key component to self-care management.
- Building a trusting relationship with your patients is essential.
- Evidence shows utilizing compassionate statements as short as 40 seconds make a meaningful difference.
- Evidence shows compassion makes a difference, with positive results for both the patient's health and the provider's.
- Evidence shows a compassionate approach reduces provider burnout.
- There is a new emerging model for health care due to advances in technology called patient-driven care.
- Patient-driven care and patient-centered care have key differences.

QUESTIONS FOR REFLECTION

- What attracted me to a nursing career?
- What approach do I take with my patients?
- Will that approach change if I am in the provider's role?
- Do I understand the difference between empathy and compassion?
- Am I willing to learn a new way of interacting with my patients?

SUGGESTED ACTIVITIES

1. Evaluate a case study and identify the areas of the nursing process at work. Look at the case and identify which stage this patient is in based on Maslow's hierarchy of needs.
2. Evaluate a case study and identify the areas of the clinical judgment model.
3. Discuss the different scopes of practice between an RN and an APRN. How are they alike and how are they different? Explore how being a nurse prepares you for becoming an APRN.
4. Discuss how the following statements make you feel:
   a. "I just need to educate my patients."
   b. "My patient is noncompliant. He just does not want to get better."
   c. "I need to find a way to motivate my patients."
   d. "It feels like a wrestling match with my patients."
5. Think of a time when you really knew someone cared about you. How did you know that? How did it make you feel?
6. Discuss the Fogarty et al. (1999) article. What are your thoughts?

References

American Association of Colleges of Nursing. (2023). *The essentials: Competencies for professional nursing education*. https://www.aacnnursing.org/Portals/0/PDFs/Publications/Essentials-2021.pdf

American Nursing Association. (2017). *The nursing process*. https://www.nursingworld.org/practice-policy/workforce/what-is-nursing/the-nursing-process

Allen, J. (2023, January 4). Understanding the 2023 Medicare hospital readmission penalty. *What I've Learned as a Hospital Medical Director*. https://hospitalmedicaldirector.com/understanding-the-2023-medicare-hospital-readmission-penalty/

Berger, B. A., & Villaume, W. A. (2019). *Motivational interviewing for health care professionals: A sensible approach* (2nd ed.). American Pharmacists Association. https://doi.org/10.21019/9781582123219.ch6

Bylund, C. L., & Makoul, G. (2005). Examining empathy in medical encounters: An observational study using the empathic communication coding system. *Health Communication, 18*(2), 123–140. https://doi.org/10.1207/s15327027hc1802_2

Dempsey, C. (2017). *The antidote to suffering: How compassionate connected care can improve safety, quality, and experience*. McGraw-Hill.

Fogarty, L. A., Curbow, B. A., Wingard, J. R., McDonnell, K., & Somerfield, M. R. (1999). Can 40 seconds of compassion reduce patient anxiety? *Journal of Clinical Oncology, 17*(1), 371–371. https://doi.org/10.1200/jco.1999.17.1.371

Martinez-Hollingsworth, A., Hicks, M., Dobrota, S. D., & Chu, L. F. (2023). Provider burnout. *Journal of Continuing Education in the Health Professions, 41*(4). https://doi.org/10.1097/ceh.0000000000000391

Roter, D. L., Hall, J. A., Kern, D. E., Barker, L. R., Cole, K. A., & Roca, R. P. (1995). Improving physicians' interviewing skills and reducing patients' emotional distress. *Archives of Internal Medicine, 155*(17), 1877–1884. https://doi.org/10.1001/archinte.1995.00430170071009

Shute, D. (2019). Motivational interviewing: Benefits and advice for busy physicians. *Contemporary OB/GYN, 64*(10), 38–40.

Swan, M. (2009). Emerging patient-driven health care models: An examination of health social networks, consumer personalized medicine and quantified self-tracking. *International Journal of Environmental Research and Public Health, 6*(2), 492–525. https://doi.org/10.3390/ijerph6020492

Trzeciak, S., & Mazzarelli, A. (2019). *Compassionomics: The revolutionary scientific evidence that caring makes a difference*. Studer Group.

Trzeciak, S., & Mazzarelli, A. (2023). *Wonder drug: 7 scientifically proven ways that serving others is the best medicine for yourself*. Essentials.

Zulman, D. M., Haverfield, M. C., Shaw, J. G., Brown-Johnson, C. G., Schwartz, R., Tierney, A. A., Zionts, D. L., Safaeinili, N., Fischer, M., Thadaney Israni, S., Asch, S. M., & Verghese, A. (2020). Practices to foster physician presence and connection with patients in the clinical encounter. *JAMA, 323*(1), 70. https://doi.org/10.1001/jama.2019.19003

Figure Credit

Fig. 3.1: Melanie Swan, "Emerging Patient-Driven Health Care Models: An Examination of Health Social Networks, Consumer Personalized Medicine and Quantified Self-Tracking," *International Journal of Environmental Research and Public Health*, vol. 6, no. 2, p. 493, MDPI. Copyright © 2009 by Melanie Swan (CC BY 3.0) at https://www.mdpi.com/1660-4601/6/2/492.

Chapter 4

Foundations of Motivational Interviewing

Motivational Interviewing is not a way of tricking people into changing; it is a way of activating their own motivation and resources for change.

—*William R. Miller*

Take a moment and think about an area in your life that you've wanted to change. It could be anything: weight loss, better time management, losing your temper less with those you love, increasing exercise, quitting smoking, eating better, being less critical of yourself or others, decreasing alcohol consumption, or any other mental or behavioral change that you've wanted to tackle. Have you felt successful in your attempts to change? If so, what approaches from others helped you the most? What approaches helped you the least? What attitudes did you encounter from your medical providers when you discussed this topic with them? Were their attitudes helpful? Were they harmful to your progress? Throughout this chapter, we will explore the processes of change, the foundations of motivational interviewing (MI), and the implications MI can have in healthcare today.

OBJECTIVES

- Students will examine the process of change through the transtheoretical theories of change model, considering how this framework supports behavior change. They will also explore the role of ambivalence as a natural part of the change process.
- Students will develop an understanding of the definitions and core principles of motivational interviewing, recognizing it as a

key component of patient-centered care.

- Students will explore the history and evolution of motivational interviewing to appreciate its development and application in practice.
- Students will identify and develop the qualities that reflect the spirit of motivational interviewing, along with the communication styles that support its effective practice.

KEY TERMS AND DEFINITIONS

- **Action:** Transtheoretical stage of change characterized by the active implementation of change strategies.
- **Ambivalence:** The state of having mixed or conflicting feelings about change, which is a central focus in MI.
- **Change:** The process through which individuals alter behaviors, habits, or thought patterns, often in response to internal motivations or external events.
- **Change talk:** In MI, statements by the patient that indicate motivation for change, including desire, ability, reasons, need, and commitment.
- **Contemplation:** The transtheoretical stage when an individual recognizes the need for change but is still ambivalent about taking action.
- **Maintenance:** The transtheoretical stage when new behaviors are sustained over time.
- **Motivational interviewing (MI):** A collaborative, person-centered counseling style designed to elicit and strengthen motivation for change by honoring autonomy and evoking internal resources.
- **Precontemplation:** The transtheoretical stage of change when an individual is not yet considering change.
- **Preparation:** The transtheoretical stage when an individual intends to act soon and begins planning for change.
- **Recycle:** A more contemporary term used in place of "relapse," emphasizing that individuals may move back into earlier stages of change and then progress forward again. Frames setbacks as a normal part of the process.
- **Relapse:** A return to previous behaviors after a period of change. Traditionally, the term "relapse" was used in the transtheoretical model to describe this process, but it has become less favored because of its negative and stigmatizing connotations. More current language uses terms such as "recycle" or "return to an earlier stage" to emphasize that setbacks are a normal part of the change process. This shift in terminology frames setbacks as opportunities for learning and growth rather than as failures.

- **Return to an earlier stage:** A neutral, descriptive phrase used in current counseling and health promotion literature to describe the process once referred to as "relapse," without the stigma associated with that term. This language underscores that behavior change is cyclical rather than linear.
- **Sustain talk:** Expressions that favor keeping things the same, indicating resistance to change.

Understanding Change

Many medical providers may have entered the field only to be surprised by how often they engage in conversations about the process of **change** with their patients. Perhaps you entered medical school or a PA or NP program expecting to focus primarily on diagnosing problems and prescribing treatments. However, in practice you've come to discover that many of your patient interactions center around guiding patients through the behavior changes they need to make but struggle to implement. Do you feel well equipped in these situations? Or do you find yourself struggling and repeating the same old advice to patients about changing habits and patterns? Is this effective?

To properly introduce the topic of **motivational interviewing (MI)**, we must first spend a bit of time talking about change—why people change and why they don't. Change may seem like a commonsense process. We've all seen patients who have had multiple heart attacks but continue to live the same lifestyle that they had before or who are resistant to take medications that have been prescribed to treat their condition. We've seen patients who have had multiple driving under influence citations (DUIs), strained relationships with family and friends, and health complications related to their substance use that still struggle to put down that drink or stop popping that pill.

Change often seems commonsensical when applied to others. It is easier to look at what others are doing and understand what they need to do to change, but it isn't as easy to look within. Change can seem simple when we apply it to others and hard when we apply it to ourselves. Think back to the questions that were posed at the beginning of the chapter. What is an area in your life for which change needs to take place? How is that going? What setbacks have you had? Have life's consequences always led to successful change? Or have consequences taken place, yet you've still found yourself turning to the same old patterns, keeping yourself locked in that familiar cycle?

Conversely, while we frequently see people grappling with change, we must also recognize that change is constantly happening. We have seen society change in marked ways after events like 9/11 or COVID, and we see people change every day. Teenagers who think they know it all mature into balanced, responsible adults. Most people, even those with serious issues like addiction, tend to move on with their lives and see improvements, without counseling intervention (Miller & Rollnick, 2002). Accidents or other events happen, and people learn to adjust. We both resist change and seek it; both things are true. What causes us to resist changing some things yet embrace it with others? The answer to that can be complex, but let's start with some of what we do know regarding why people change.

Change Is Natural

First, change is natural. Miller and Rollnick (2002) discuss in their book *Motivational Interviewing: Preparing People for Change* that while we think that change can only begin after we as the experts have initiated it, change takes place just as often when a person does not receive treatment. Many smokers or problem gamblers make positive life changes whether they receive formal treatment or not. We used to think of these "spontaneous recoveries" as rare events, but that is not the case. In fact, we have learned that individuals who recover go through the same processes with or without treatment. Treatment can aid in the process, but we as health care providers can facilitate this change with our patients just by being attentive to it.

Brief Interactions Can Be Impactful

Often, we think that we must work with a patient for a long time to see "real" change take place, but what we have learned from research is that often a person can begin to change from just one interaction, if the conditions are right (Miller & Rollnick, 2002). When we take the time, even in a one-time patient encounter, to establish a collaborative, nonjudgmental working relationship with our patients, we can make an impact. We can build trust and rapport that might lead us forward in a positive direction with other sessions or lay the groundwork for future insight and change. Patients who have experienced an interaction with a provider that was supportive, open, affirming, and empowering may be more likely to seek out additional help later. Even a one-time encounter can be a potentially transformative experience.

Faith and Hope Matter for Change

What one believes one achieves. When we think we can change we are much more likely to do so. When you ask a patient how likely they think they are to be able to initiate a change in behavior, their answer is highly indicative of that outcome (Miller & Rollnick, 2002). The concept of self-efficacy has to do with whether a person believes that they can change. One thing that can shape self-efficacy is belief (or lack thereof) from others around us. If a provider communicates that they believe in us, that creates an environment where the patient can internalize that provider's belief and use it to create a sense of belief in themselves. This means that we need to counter our own biases in thinking that certain patients are noncompliant or too far gone or whatever else we might tell ourselves and start to see that our patients *can* change. Let our belief be so strong that the patient can feel it from us because our belief in them supports the impetus of their change. We can be their biggest supporters.

Provider-Specific Effects Support Change

I used to go through the local McDonald's drive through to get a Diet Coke regularly, and I started to notice that on the days when one employee took my order I felt much happier after the encounter than on others. No matter who served me, I would still get that crispy Diet Coke to start my day, but her warmth, friendliness, and conveyance of care for me in those brief interactions really brightened my day compared to other employees who helped me on other days. I found myself feeling disappointed when she wasn't working. We can all think of instances like this when it wasn't what someone did for us but *how* they did it that made all the difference. We are finding this to be more and more true in health care. It is true that the way someone interacts with patients makes all the difference. We will discuss this more when we learn about Carl Rogers in the next chapter, along with other humanistic approaches, but for now it is important to note that research supports that the impact of provider-specific traits has a positive impact on behavior change outcomes for patients.

Just take the quality of empathy as one example. Providers who demonstrate empathy in their patient encounters have had increased health outcomes for patients and higher overall patient satisfaction rates (Derksen et al., 2013; Surchat et al., 2022). Patients want to be seen as people first. They want to know that their providers care. There is a timeless saying often attributed to Theodore Roosevelt: "People need to know how much you care, before they care how much you know." This is true in many situations, and it is especially so in health care when patients come to us in some of their most vulnerable moments in life. Who the provider is and how they interact with their patients truly does matter.

There are many factors that influence and support change, and understanding the stages of change is an important way to help us understand where and how our motivational interviewing strategies can be applied. To do so, let's discuss the transtheoretical stages of change model.

The Transtheoretical Stages of Change

The transtheoretical stages of change (TSC) model helps us understand that change is a process. It outlines the stages of readiness that individuals go through as they prepare for change. By actively listening to our patients, we can begin to recognize their current state of readiness for change. The TSC model was created by Prochaska and DiClemente in 1983; they applied it when working with smokers who wanted to quit. They believed that once practitioners could identify a patient's readiness for change, they could apply techniques that matched that level of change and see more success from patients. The stages of change are outlined as follows:

1. **Precontemplation**: Individual is not ready for change.
2. **Contemplation**: Individual has begun to see a need for change.
3. **Preparation**: Individual expects to change in the next month or so.
4. **Action**: Individual is actively implementing a plan to change.
5. **Maintenance**: Individual has engaged in at least 6 months of the action phase.
6. Termination: Individual has successfully changed their behavior.

"**Recycle**" or "**return to an earlier stage**," formerly known as "**relapse**," most often occurs between the action and maintenance stages. The stages of change are not linear; individuals may enter and reenter them many times. Because sustaining change is challenging, recycling or returning to an earlier stage should not be viewed as failure but as a normal part of the process. This shift in terminology reflects a more supportive, cyclical view of behavior change. By using open-ended questions, empathy, and collaboration, providers can better assess where a patient is in their journey and apply MI strategies appropriate to that stage (Dixon et al., 2023; Prochaska & DiClemente, 1983).

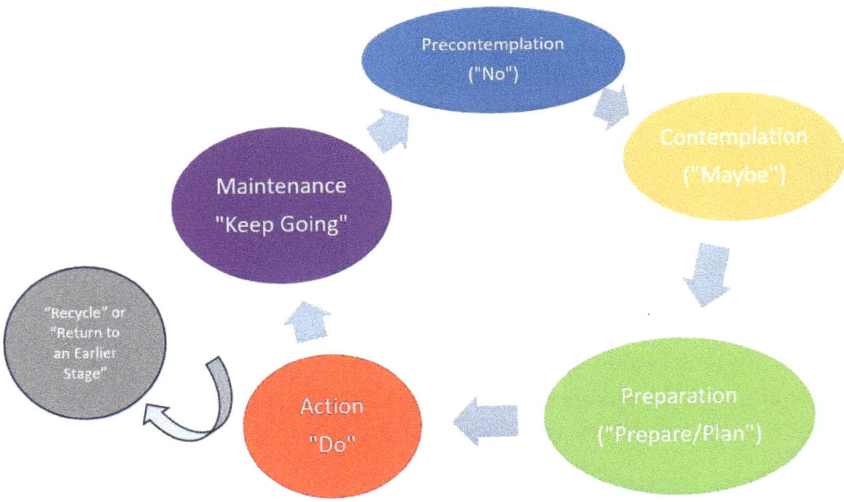

Figure 4.1 Transtheoretical Stages of Change

Let's look at how an individual facing the issue of smoking might express themselves at each stage of change, along with the corresponding provider response that aligns with each stage.

1. Precontemplation

   Patient: "I don't think I have a problem. Smoking helps me relax, and I don't see a reason to quit."

   Provider: "It sounds like smoking is one thing that you can rely on to help you relax. You don't see a reason to quit. Often people find that something helps them in one way but harms them in others. Would you be open to talking about any of the ways that smoking doesn't serve you?"

2. Contemplation

   Patient: "I know I should probably quit smoking someday, but I'm not sure I am ready yet."

   Provider: "It sounds like you do see a need to quit smoking and plan to work toward that one day. What are some of the reasons that you feel the need to quit?"

3. Preparation

   Patient: "I've been thinking about cutting back, and I'm planning to quit next month, but I'm worried it might be too hard."

   Provider: "It sounds like you have been thinking about cutting back and are ready to make a plan, but you worry about how challenging the process will be. What are some of the challenges that you anticipate, and what has helped you get through tough situations in the past?"

4. Action

   Patient: "I stopped smoking last week, but it's really tough. I'm craving cigarettes all the time."

   Provider: "It sounds like you have been able to stop smoking for about a week. That is wonderful. It sounds like you are having success, but it is also still really hard for you. What have you done that has helped you through your cravings so far?"

5. Maintenance

   Patient: "I've been smoke-free for 6 months now, but every once in a while, I think about having a cigarette."

   Provider: "That's a really big accomplishment! Six months smoke free is not easy. It is completely normal to have thoughts about smoking occasionally.

What has helped you to stay on track and resist the urges when the thoughts and cravings come? And how do you feel when you look back at how far you've come? How has your life changed?"

6. Recycle or return to an earlier stage

   Patient: "I tried to quit but started smoking again last month. I feel like I've failed."

   Provider: "It sounds like you made an attempt to quit smoking, and you started up again, which leaves you feeling like you've failed. It is understandable to be disappointed with yourself when you have a setback, but this is not a failure. It is part of the process for many people. What do you think you've learned from this experience that might help you next time?"

Listening for these types of statements can help providers determine where their patient is at on their change journey so that they can respond appropriately. These responses meet the patient where they are. They establish that this is a collaborative relationship. They express compassion, evoke **change talk**, and empower the patient to keep trying. How does reading these exchanges make you feel? How do you think you would respond to these statements currently? Do you feel that your responses are already in line with this type of thinking, or is this a chance for you to begin to shift your thinking? How would you describe your current stage in the change process when it comes to reflecting on your growth as a provider and your willingness to adopt the MI model? As we contemplate embracing a new way to interact with patients, we actually go through the stages of change ourselves. Now that we've discussed the TSC model, let's talk about MI and how we can use it to support the change process.

The Birth of Motivational Interviewing

MI was developed in the early 1980s by William R. Miller and Stephen Rollnick, clinical psychologists who have worked in the field of addiction. When MI was developed, many of the prevailing approaches to working with individuals struggling with substance use were confrontational. The belief was that the individual needed to face their addiction head on and overcome it. Thus, many working with this population used confrontational and challenging approaches that were meant to break individuals down to lead to a "breakthrough," which would lead to change. While these methods may have been useful for some, for many they did more harm than good. When confronted, individuals often became defensive and resistant to change. Instead of these methods motivating people to change, in many cases it caused them to pull away even further.

Miller saw opportunities for introducing a new approach while working in Norway. While there, he noticed that clinicians interacted with patients in ways that encouraged them to broaden their thinking and become more open to change. Many people are ambivalent when it comes to change. One part of them wants to lean in and change their behavior, while another part feels scared, uncertain, or resistant. Miller noticed that patients responded better when they were met with empathy and collaboration. He built on the humanistic, person-centered theory of psychotherapy put forth by Carl Rogers and applied it to the field of addiction, and this led to the birth of MI. Miller believed, like Rogers, that people respond better to therapists who approach them with an attitude of respect and a desire to understand rather than to confront, coerce, or lecture. Miller understood that when we approach people with respect, nonjudgment, and empathy we allow them to lead and facilitate an environment where self-reflection is encouraged and openness to change blossoms.

Person-centered therapy embodies the idea that the patient, not the provider, is the expert of their lives. Providers do not walk through the day-to-day interactions and complexities that the patient does. Providers do not know the full history or look at the world through the exact lens that patients do. Thus, providers must acknowledge that within the patient lies an expertise that we can never attain. Person-centered therapy believes that if we create the right environment and embody an authentic, empathic presence, a person will know what to do for their lives. Rogers developed three key conditions that therapists must possess to facilitate a patient's growth: empathy, unconditional positive regard, and congruence (also known as genuineness). These concepts will be explored in depth in Chapter 5. Applying these Rogerian conditions, along with techniques that draw out and build upon a person's own internal motivation for change, is the heart of MI.

Miller and Rollnick formalized their approach in the 1980s and wrote their first book on MI in 1991, titled *Motivational Interviewing: Preparing People to Change Addictive Behavior.* Miller and Rollnick (2023) discuss the selection of the name for their approach, pointing out that they did so because motivation is what gets someone going. It is what leads to change. They feel that no one is unmotivated, but they also feel that sometimes people need help tapping into their motivations and drawing them forward. They mention that they selected the word "interviewing" to indicate that the interviewer has a certain role that goes beyond that of just a conversation; they are also tasked with guiding the conversation forward. The interviewer could be a person who asks questions to determine who to hire for a job, but they could also be a student asked to interview someone for an assignment. Either way, the interviewer needs to be a curious, motivated, active listener who knows how to ask questions in a way that can evoke compelling and useful responses that help us understand the person that they are talking to. Miller and Rollnick (2023) emphasize that they did not select the term "motivational interviewing" because the interviewer instills motivation into the person. Rather, they draw out motivation that is already there.

MI is a conversational approach that engages the patient to meet them where they are and allow them to be a part of finding their own path forward. Practitioners who use MI work on building therapeutic rapport that will allow the patient to investigate their own **ambivalence** regarding the feelings that they hold toward change and find solutions themselves (Rollnick et al., 2008). Ambivalence is common when it comes to change. Rarely does one decide to change and never waver in that decision. We may want to be on time for work but still cling to those few extra minutes of sleep in the morning as we continue to hit the snooze button. We may want to make time for walking 30 minutes a day but find ourselves wanting to sit on the couch as soon as we get in the door after a hard day at work. How can we lean into these feelings of ambivalence, allow ourselves to hold two truths at once, and work our way toward a solution?

MI can help. Traditionally, when a person has a health concern they go to their provider. The provider is tasked with asking a set of questions, coming to a diagnostic conclusion, and prescribing a course of treatment (Rollnick et al., 2008). This is what many patients have come to expect, and this is what providers hold the responsibility to do. The problem with this approach is two-fold. One, it does not involve the patient in the solution. This means that the patient may or may not be able to follow through with what is prescribed. Two, it places a hefty weight on providers: Not only must they use their medical training and expertise to diagnose what is going on medically, but they feel solely responsible for health outcomes when patients may not be able to follow through with their plans. This can lead to burnout on the part of providers who feel that they are not making a difference.

One foundational principle of MI is exploring and building on the patient's own motivation to see what will work for them. Perhaps a patient has elevated blood glucose levels, and a provider wants to prescribe them a strict diet to cut out all extra carbs and sugars. Would this be helpful to their health outcome? Perhaps, but is this patient ready for such a drastic change? Maybe not. If the provider can engage in a conversation with the patient, they can see what areas the patient is ready to change. Perhaps they aren't ready to change everything all at once, but maybe they are motivated to use a food journal to start monitoring what they are eating. Perhaps they are willing to switch from full-sugar soda to diet. Engaging the patient helps them to feel in control, and it allows nonjudgement, acceptance, and celebration of small successes to become part of the provider-patient relationship. This might seem small, but it is not. It is one of the biggest keys to the MI approach.

Think of your own medical experiences. Have there been times when you needed to go to the doctor, but you put it off because you knew that you had not made the lifestyle changes that they would want to hear? We can change these interactions by creating a space where patients feel safe to share successes *and setbacks* without fear of judgment. Creating this space is something that I call "the sacred space" (Dixon et al., 2023). We often think of religion when the term "sacred" is used. The term connotes something special, precious, safe, and connected to God or a spiritual leader. However, in this context we are talking about a space where the patient can feel completely free to be open, vulnerable, and safe with their provider.

Providers have come to term patients who have not met the planned goals as unmotivated for change "noncompliant" or "difficult", but patients have simply seen the progress for their health *differently* than the provider. When we encounter patients like this, providers may feel as if they have failed or that the patient is unwilling to make the necessary changes in their life to be healthy. They may even write them off, feeling that there is nothing more they can do. This is not the case. Rollnick et al. (2008) state that "change is actually quite malleable and is particularly formed in the context of relationships" (p. 6). How we talk to and interact with our patients does impact their outcomes. This leads us into the "spirit" of MI.

The Spirit of Motivational Interviewing

So much of what MI is goes beyond merely techniques; it is who we are as providers and how we approach our patients. How do we view them? Do we have a sense of curiosity about what is happening with them? Do we care about their stories and view them with empathy? Do we care to understand what motivates them and view them as individuals who oversee their own lives, including their own health care? What is more personal to someone than their own body? Their own health? The spirit of MI is made up of the four guiding principles of partnership, acceptance, compassion, and empowerment (Miller & Rollnick, 2023).

Partnership

The first principle within the spirit of MI is partnership. Partnership means that instead of a one-up, one-down relationship, the patient and provider work together as equals. Conversations are collaborative, and decisions are made together. This type of relationship is essential in health care because ultimately the patient is the one responsible for behavior change outcomes. Partnership means *coming alongside your patients* and finding a balance between directing and following the patient (Miller & Rollnick, 2023). When we direct, we tell people that x, y, and z need to happen, and they need to do it this way. Think of a movie set with the director telling an actor to show more emotion. When we follow, it is a passive process. Think of the game follow the leader. It can be fun, but we aren't involved in the decisions. We mimic the next movement selected by the leader. With MI we don't want to direct, and we don't want to follow. Instead, we are more like tour guides. We know the city, but we want to show our tour group things on the tour that they want to see. Say we are in Rome. There is a lot to see in Rome that the tour guide is familiar with and could show the tour group, but knowing if the tour group is more interested in historical sites, food and culture, or art would allow for the guide to most effectively plan a week of adventure that the tour group would benefit the most from. The same is true with MI in health care. We are experts in our field. We are the cardiologist. We are the psychiatric nurse practitioner, or primary care DO. We have expertise in our field, but we partner with our patients in a way that allows them to decide what happens, based on their situation, and we guide them along their chosen path, providing information and evoking information from patients to help us do so.

Acceptance

Acceptance means that the provider respects, values, and supports the patient as they are, without judgment, and this acceptance is *not* conditional upon the patient's willingness to change. This is difficult. When a patient does not want to do what we prescribe, we may view accepting that as a failure on our part. However, when we demonstrate acceptance and understanding, we are not failing the patient. We are demonstrating to them that we are there with them, no matter what, and when they see this, they may be more willing to engage in "change talk."

Another part of acceptance is honoring autonomy, which means that we learn to take a step back. We convey an understanding that the patient is in charge. Everyone is allowed to make their own choices. We can educate, share our expertise, and inform patients how certain behaviors may impact their health outcomes, but ultimately it is up to them in what they choose to do. This can be difficult. Most of us who go into helping professions do so because we want to help or even "save" people, so when we encounter patients who are not willing or are not able to implement sustained change behaviors, we take it personally. However, we must acknowledge that there is only so much that we can control, but—and this is a big "but"—we can promise to be there with our patients no matter what, even when they miss the mark. Our acceptance of them is unconditional. In fact, in the field of psychotherapy there is a concept called unconditional positive regard. Carl Rogers put forth this idea that we must have an attitude of complete acceptance of our patients. With this approach, we don't judge; we accept, and we understand their story and their autonomy without rejection or criticism. Again, this does not mean that we lie or pretend that certain behaviors will not negatively impact our patients' health, but we acknowledge that they have the freedom to make changes or not to. Rollnick et al. (2008) state, "Ironically, it is acknowledging the other's right and freedom not to change that sometimes makes change possible" (p. 7).

Compassion

The third principle embodied within the spirit of MI is compassion. We need to truly care and want our patients to do well. We need to act in ways that demonstrate beneficence in their lives. Beneficence means to do good, and we are all familiar with this principle. None of us went into health care, whether physical health or mental health, wanting to do harm. We understand that compassion means serving our patients with kindness, to stand by their side as they face some of their hardest moments. Compassion is science with a soul, creating that sacred space where patients can feel truly comfortable with us because they know they are cared for no matter what. To do good for our patients and to put empathy into action, using the principle of compassion, we must step into our patients' worlds enough that we understand what they think would make it better. Is it an aggressive health care plan and treatment? Is it being able to stabilize their oxygen levels enough that they can go on a nightly walk with their partner each day, even if they aren't ready to fully quit smoking? Is it something else? We know what will improve medical conditions, but we don't know what our patients are ready for. We don't know what they need. We need to care enough, to be compassionate enough that we let them tell us, and then we help them find their way forward.

Empowerment

When we realize that it is not our job to "do" something to our patients, it is our job to evoke skills, strengths, and motivations from within them so that they can do what they want to do given the expertise that we've shared and the relationship we've created, we embody the principle of empowerment. We want them to understand that they took charge of their health care. They took steps to create the behavior changes that they decided to embark upon. It was not us who did it for or to them; we just helped them understand all their options. They made the choice. They made the change. Think back on your life to times when you relied on others to do something for you, but then you were empowered to do it for yourself, such as learning to ride a bike, taking off the training wheels, and perhaps falling a few times, but with support from a loved one seeing that you had the strength. You could keep trying and do it yourself. We can empower our patients in the same ways. We can help them chunk progress into steps and see what they can do and what they are willing to do to get a better outcome. Maybe they aren't great at checking their blood sugar levels several times a day as instructed, but maybe they are willing to set a timer on their phone so that they can check it once daily. We can empower them to take ownership and decide the next steps based on their skills and strengths.

Often when we convey partnership, acceptance, compassion, and an attitude of empowerment for our patients we can help them to put down their defenses and consider their situation more openly. It may surprise you, but often when we establish this collaborative relationship it frees the patient to lean into change rather than to resist our efforts to make them do so. This is not done as a game or some type of reverse psychology in that we are trying to "trick" our patients into doing what we view as right, but it is an opportunity for us to establish a relationship with them that allows changes to look different than we thought. Think of a patient with lung cancer who is still smoking. We tell them that they need to quit immediately, even when they are not ready to do so. That can put a barrier in our relationship that doesn't allow either of us to get what we need from this interaction. We can't change their mind, and they don't feel like they can get help until they can please us by meeting our demands. If we approach this differently, we could discuss their prognosis and situation while also exploring their goals and hopes within this context. By doing so, we could collaborate to implement small changes that still have a positive impact on their health. Maybe they could cut back on smoking. Maybe there are treatments that we could still offer that would be more effective if they were to fully stop smoking, but by still offering those treatments maybe they could find an alleviation of symptoms to still have enough oxygen to be able to continue to go on nightly walks with their partner. This is still a positive health change, and we must start to see as providers that even small changes may be huge for our patients. Even mental shifts and small alterations in how patients think can be progress, or maybe we will see how smoking helps our patients cope with the anxiety of having lung cancer and all that entails and accept them where they are.

A story that showed me the importance of celebrating small changes came when working with a woman who was participating in treatment court (Dixon et al., 2023). I met with her for our weekly one-on-one counseling appointment, and I asked her how she was doing. She replied by telling me that she had given up her belt. Unsure of what that meant, I sat there with her for a moment. Then I asked her to tell me more. She went on to tell me that she had thrown away the belt that she used to tie off with before she injected heroin. For many, this might appear to be a small victory worth a bit of celebration, but they may not truly grasp the significance of what this step meant for her.

I allowed her to elaborate on what the belt meant to her and how big of a sacrifice that this "small" step was given her circumstances. The belt was a reminder that caused her cravings to intensify, so letting it go was a big deal. However, many participants in the treatment court, herself included, struggle tremendously with economic stability. She was paying for a room in a shared housing unit with temporary vouchers that had been issued to her by a foundation that supports the treatment court while she looked for a job that would work around her treatment court obligations. She did not have transportation, and she did not have money for groceries, let alone another belt that she could use to hold up her pants that were way too big for her at the time. As I looked at her, I noticed that she held her pants up with a piece of rope that she tied around them. Still, she was willing to let go of something that was literally helping hold herself together because she wanted to embrace change that badly.

I would love to say that I know that she was able to successfully complete treatment court and go forward to reach every one of her dreams. Unfortunately, I do not know the full outcome of her story. I do know that I worked with her in treatment court for another few weeks, and she and a few other participants ended up all relapsing because they decided to try "bath salts" together. I know this led to some jail time for them, but I am uncertain of how things have turned out for her today. I certainly wish her the best, and I am so thankful for my short time with her because it showed me how important it is to really listen and understand the journey that our patients are on.

For many who have stable income, access to clothing, food, and other necessities of life it may be hard to understand the struggle. We may look at someone like this woman and think that her return to use reflects noncompliance or a lack of motivation. In reality, one part of her wanted change so much that she was willing to give up something that helped hold herself together, while another part, shaped by complex biological, psychological, social, and environmental factors, could not sustain change at this time. We need to be ready to meet our patients on the day that they announce that they have given up their belts and on the day that they return after serving a court sanction related to their return to use. Our role is to stand with them regardless.

Four Tasks of MI

In addition to the four guiding principles that make up the spirit of MI, Miller and Rollnick (2023) describe four tasks that we must keep in mind to guide patients toward conversations related to behavior change. These tasks help us to increase "change talk," explore their motivations, and resolve ambivalence to change.

Figure 4.2 Four Tasks of MI

The first task in MI is called engaging. This is a foundational task and will continue to be used throughout the use of the three other tasks: focusing, evoking, and planning. When we engage with patients, we work to create a working alliance with them. Miller and Rollnick (2023) state that there is solid evidence to support that creating a positive working relationship with patients leads to opportunities when change can take place. How can we establish a good working alliance? We can start by exhibiting the principles outlined in the spirit of MI. We want to build a collaborative relationship in which we have established trust and created rapport with the patient. We want them to feel comfortable talking to us. We want to demonstrate that they are in a safe place, and we won't judge them. We want to show them that we've created a space where open conversations can take place. We want to hear what they have to say, and we want to use active listening techniques to demonstrate that we are listening and show we do understand. The essential question that Miller and Rollnick (2023) say we are asking of patients in the engage phase is "Can we walk together?" We don't have to know where we are going just yet, but do we want them to feel safe with us in this journey? Do they trust us to guide them?

Once we've established this, the next task is focusing. In this phase the questions become "Where are we going?" and "What are we going to talk about?" (Miller & Rollnick, 2023, p. 23). In the focus phase, we help the patient identify a clear direction. Miller and Rollnick (2023) state that while MI is not directive in the sense that we tell patients what to do, it is directional. We interact with them in ways that help the patient identify and clarify a specific goal or change. We help them explore and resolve ambivalence. We work to narrow the scope and define priorities and values, and we explore whether their current actions align with the values and priorities that the patient has identified. As helpers we often want to direct the focus and prescribe change, but this is not effective. We cannot make people change, no matter how clearly we tell them. Thus, in MI we are not prescribing goals. We are sharing goals, and a goal doesn't become a goal until the patient agrees to it. In fact, goals are best when the patient is the one who identifies them.

To help patients get to the point that they can identify goals, we must learn to embrace the third task of MI, evoking. Miller and Rollnick (2023) say that the underlying question with this task is "Why would you go there?" (p. 24). Evoking is when we really start to target ambivalence to change. We've discussed ambivalence already, the idea that often when we approach a situation for which we want change to take place, there are just as many reasons for us to not want to change as there are for us to want to change. We may want to get in better shape, but we also want to relax when we come home from work instead of going to the gym. MI acknowledges this push–pull happens within us all, and this is when interviewing skills can help us to either evoke, or elicit, change talk. Change talk is when the patient talks about the motivations or positive steps they want to take or are taking toward the change. There is also **sustain talk**, which is when the patient talks about things that move them away from change and continue things as they are. We want to decrease sustain talk and offer ample opportunities for the patient to discuss change talk. As the "interviewers" we can influence whether change talk or sustain talk takes place through the questions we ask and don't ask and through the summaries and reflections we make and don't make. We want to talk in ways that give the patient plenty of time to talk about thoughts toward change, steps toward change, and actions that indicate changes are taking place. For example, if a patient comes in and says that they didn't stick to their diet or exercise goals much but did manage to pack their lunch instead of eating fast food, you can ask about that one small change. Build on that. Even if they report that they have done nothing at all since their last appointment, evoking does sometimes involve the provider evoking hope, evoking optimism, and evoking belief that the patient can change and can do this in the future, even if they are not ready now.

The last task of MI is planning. Miller and Rollnick (2023) teach that the task of planning moves us from talking about why we would want to walk to where we are walking to "how will you get there?" (p. 25). Providers need to continue to rely on the skills that they used in engaging, focusing, and evoking. We need to engage the person in the planning. We need their help to focus on what is important for them, for they hold the answers to what is most important in their lives. We need to evoke answers from within them about what plan would work. Operating from within the MI framework means that the provider understands that they should not be imposing a plan because they do not have all the information and expertise to do so. Yes, they do have medical expertise, but the patient is the expert on their lives. They are the ones who must create and accept the plan because they will have to carry it out. We can help patients by evoking change talk that helps the patient to create a realistic and actionable plan that includes small, achievable steps toward their goal. We can create discussions that strengthen their commitment to the changes that they have decided to embark upon. We can help support them and strengthen them in their follow-through because of the collaborative, supportive relationship that we have created with them. We must also remember that planning is not a one-and-done session. It is ongoing. Plans are made. Plans are changed. One goal may be achieved, and then we focus on another, or we may decide to hold off on one goal to work on another.

Rollnick et al. (2008) use the acronym RULE to teach these four principles. The R stands for resisting the righting reflex. The U stands for understanding and exploring the patient's own motivations. The L stands for listening with empathy, and the E stands for empowering the patient, encouraging hope and optimism.

Resist the Righting Reflex

Resisting the righting reflex and learning to roll with resistance can be very difficult for health care providers. Nurses entering advanced practice training many times feel the answer to all their patient's woes is to educate them on the correct health choices. The internal desire to right a wrong or impart our expert knowledge is ever present, and we find it difficult to know how to take another approach. Our desire to help or educate is not bad. It often stems from a desire to help, guide, and prevent negative health outcomes for patients, but when we take on a lecturing or persuading approach the natural reaction from many patients is to resist. It is to "yes, but" in response. Just think back to our teenage years. How often were our parents right? Yet, how often were we ready to hear it? This impulse to resist can be particularly strong when we are already ambivalent about the change.

For example, many who are facing addiction know it is a problem for them. Many want to change, but they also enjoy the way that they feel after having a drink to loosen up with friends socially or after smoking a cigarette upon getting home after a long day. It can be instinctive for people to want to argue the opposite when presented with someone who is trying to tell them that their behaviors are causing problems in their lives. This can even lead to a power struggle between the provider and the patient, and we know once we enter a power struggle no one has "won." Think of a time when you tried to talk to a patient. Maybe you were telling them that this antidepressant medication would help alleviate their symptoms, and they responded by saying, "Well, my depression isn't too bad. I don't think I need to start taking something." Then we try to convince them further, and they get more defensive, offer more reasons not to, and so on.

Rollnick et al. (2008) point out that no matter how good a provider's medical arguments are for change they cannot surpass the role of human nature. We tend to resist an argument that someone else is making, but we tend to listen to our own voices and build on our own reasons for change. To use these facts to our advantage we can change how we talk with our patients. Instead of us lecturing them on what they should do, and meeting their "but this" and "but that" responses with more counterarguments that continue this back and forth, we can roll with their resistance and begin to put them in the role of exploring solutions. Let them talk it out and build on what they say. For most often, the problem that impedes the patient making necessary changes is not a lack of knowledge; it is ambivalence. We can work with this ambivalence when we don't resist resistance, and we can deepen our conversations with patients by implementing the remainder of the letters in the RULE acronym.

Understand Your Patient's Motives

With the MI approach, providers use the patient's reasons for change to drive the path forward (Rollnick et al., 2008). They don't simply impose their own ideas onto their patients. This requires creating a foundation of understanding. It requires tossing out the old, medical model approach and asking questions in a way that gets the patient to do most of the talking. Providers need to get patients talking about their concerns and motivations so that they can be explored and built upon. Instead of thinking of ourselves as teachers who are educating patients, we can begin thinking of ourselves as guides. Think of yourself as a travel guide. When you work with a patient, you want to get to know them well enough to understand how they like to travel and the destinations that they want to see. This allows you to work with them to plan for a destination. You would present various travel package options, you would point out the pros and cons with each package, and you would ask them which option makes the most sense to them. Then, you would listen and allow them the freedom to choose which option works for them without judging their choice.

The biggest fear for many providers when it comes to implementing this principle is how much time it could take. However, we have found that this can be done and done effectively even in short patient encounters. Rollnick et al. (2008) say that time spent asking the patient why they want to make a change and exploring how they might go about doing so is the best way to spend our time with patients when time is limited. Creating opportunities for discussion around change, or change talk, is at the heart of MI. Change talk leads to change, and the patient's own voice discussing and exploring options for change will be the most impactful. We will share more techniques for how to do this in Chapter 6.

Listen to Your Patient

Listening is a complex skill. You may have heard the following platitudes regarding listening: "We were given two ears and one mouth for a reason," or "We need to listen to understand and not to respond." Platitudes usually become such because they contain wisdom that resonates with people. These sayings are true, and the art of listening is one that counselors-in-training spend several classes learning how to do well. It sounds like a simple skill, but effective listening is broken up into complex parts.

- *Attending:* Attending is made up of several parts that make up the way we demonstrate our presence. Attending includes our physical presence. It includes being fully present, using open body language, and maintaining eye contact that conveys a sense of empathy and attentiveness.
- *Understanding:* To demonstrate understanding, we must demonstrate empathy, ask open-ended questions to make sure we have fully comprehended the speaker's message, and master the art of summary and paraphrase to indicate that we've fully taken in and understand the speaker's message.
- *Reflection:* Reflection involves mirroring back our patient's feelings by acknowledging the emotional content of their message and validating their feelings and perspective.
- *Responding:* Knowing how to respond in a way that encourages the speaker to elaborate is important with motivational interviewing. This can be done using both verbal and nonverbal encouragers (e.g., "I see," or "go on," "that makes sense," or nodding, smiling, leaning in toward the patient, raising eyebrows, etc.). Responding also includes asking thoughtful questions that convey genuine interest and invite deeper exploration, as well as providing constructive, empathic feedback that does not convey judgment.
- *Remembering:* One of the best ways to convey that we are listening is being able to recall key points and details of what someone has shared with you. We can do this by referencing things that patients have shared with us earlier in the visit or from previous appointments.

These are just some of the components involved in active listening. It is a extremely complex clinical skill that counselors, social workers, psychologists, and others in the field of mental health and communications specialties spend a great deal of time and training on. This is not mentioned to put undue pressure on providers or for anyone to feel the need to be perfect at this skill or any of the others stressed in this book, but it is important to remember that even when we listen to a patient, very important work *is* happening. We are making strides, developing rapport, and realizing that when we are talking about behavior change, the answers come from within the patient, and to find them we must learn to listen.

Empower Your Patient

Empowering patients is one of the most important aspects of the MI approach. When we empower patients in the process, we help them take ownership by honoring their autonomy. Patients are also much more likely to follow through with change steps when they are the ones to generate the actions. Our role shifts from prescriber of solutions to facilitator of discovery. We learn to ask questions in ways that will draw out the answers from the expert source, our patients. We still share our expertise, we discuss the pluses and minuses of various approaches, but we ask them to decide which path to take to carry out the changes that they need for themselves. When we empower our patients, we help them to see that they are in charge of their health. They learn a new way of thinking about their own health and wellness that they can continue to apply throughout their lives.

Communication Styles in MI

Learning to embody the spirit of MI can seem simple on the surface, but it is quite complex. It takes practice to find the right balance among guiding, directing, and following your patients. Rollnick et al. (2008) talk about how MI should feel like a dance with your patients rather than a wrestling match. We must balance three communication styles in our interactions with patients: following, directing, and guiding.

Following

When we implement the following approach to communication, we primarily rely on the skill of listening. We follow the direction of the conversation. The message that we convey when we use this method is "I trust you. I know you will find the answer in your own way at your own time." There are times in patient encounters when this is appropriate. For example, when you first start working with a patient, using a period of following can help you understand the patient's symptoms, how they feel, or what they need. Another time when the following approach is useful is after delivering difficult news to a patient. They need time to process their feelings, and we can allow them this space to do so, without judgment, just following along their journey of emotion.

Directing

There are times when we need a director, someone who is clearly in charge and can share their expertise. This type of communication is common in medical provider training programs, and there are times when it is the right approach to take. Situations when the patient needs to know what to do for their safety come to mind. Many patients come to you because they want this approach, so it does have its place. When we communicate in a directive style, we let the patient know, "I know what you need to do. I have knowledge that can help you in this area. You can trust my expertise." However, just like everything, direction needs to have its place, and when applied at the wrong time, it can detract from a patient's progress.

Guiding

What is the difference between directing and guiding? Those terms seem similar, but there are differences. A director tells you what to do. A guide leads you. A guide gives you resources that can help you find your path. A tour guide wants to know your interests so that they can plan the right trip, highlight key points of knowledge that are meaningful to you along the way. When we communicate with the guiding style, we convey the message "I can help you decide where you want to go. I can provide knowledge that will help you make the best healthcare decisions for you."

We need to find the right blend for these approaches. We don't want to be all follower, all guide, or all director. We need to be flexible and open and always assess where our patients are and how we can meet them in that journey. It may be helpful to ask ourselves, "If I were in this situation, would I want someone to follow me and hear me out, would I want someone to tell me which way to go, or would I want someone to provide insight and help guide me down a path that I create for myself?" Overly relying on one method or the other can create challenges with our patients.

Change Talk

One of the key concepts in MI is listening for and evoking what is known as change talk. Change talk refers to the things that someone says that signal a desire, ability, or commitment to make a change in their behavior. This can look different for each person, depending on which stage of change they are in. If they aren't there yet, that's okay. You can still talk with them about it by expressing empathy, asking open-ended questions, using reflective listening, eliciting their perspectives, exploring hypotheticals, and gently developing discrepancies.

The concepts associated with change talk can be explained using the acronym DARN-CAT (Miller & Rollnick, 2023):

1. Desire: Look for expressions of wanting or wishing for change.
    - Example: "I want to stop drinking."
2. Ability: Look for statements from the patient regarding their capability to change.

- Example: "I think I can do this."

3. Reasons: Listen for specific reasons that your patient wants to change.
    - Example: "I really want to exercise so that I can feel healthy again."
4. Need: Statements related to the urgency associated with change taking place made by the patient.
    - Example: "I have to get healthier so that I can be there for my kids."
5. Commitment: Expressions by the patient of intent or decision to act.
    - Example: "I will start eating healthier tomorrow."
6. Activation: Indicates that a patient is ready to act.
    - Example: "I'm ready to sign up for the program."
7. Taking steps: Statements made by the patient that they have been taking actions already.
    - Example: "I've started cutting back on cigarettes."

Importance of Change Talk

Change talk is important because it works on those feelings of ambivalence that are part of change and allows the patient to talk freely with a person who wants to help them connect with their own internal motivations for change. Change talk is an essential element of MI because

- it increases the person's motivation for change;
- it reflects their ambivalence shifting toward change;
- it supports the likelihood of them acting.

The opposite of change talk is called sustain talk, which is when the patient expresses resistance to change or a desire for things to stay the same. What we talk about we create, so we want to get patients engaged in more change talk and less sustain talk. Sustain talk can sound like this:

- "I don't really want to quit smoking."
- "I don't think I can lose weight. I've tried before, and I always gain it back."
- "Drinking helps me relax after a hard day at work."
- "I don't have time to exercise."
- "I'm just not ready to give it up yet."

When we hear sustain talk, we don't need to fight against it. This gives us a lot of information about where our patient is in their thought process. We can learn not to feed into our "fix it" and "resist it" instinct when we hear sustain talk and learn not to respond by offering opposing opinions or advice by looking at sustain talk as information that can help us understand our patients. We can let our defenses down and learn to respond by acknowledging the patient's concerns in a nonjudgmental way, exploring their ambivalence on the issue. It is likely that even if they aren't ready to give it up yet, a part of them understands that they need to. We could respond to a statement such as "Drinking helps me to relax after work" by saying, "On one hand it sounds like drinking helps you to relax, but on the other hand, I know you're also worried about your health." This would allow for them to share and explore their feelings on both sides and for you to talk about the pros and cons of changing their behavior. You can also shift the focus of the conversation by redirecting them back to strengths that they have or previous successes that they've shared. You might remind them "You mentioned before that you felt better when you exercised. Tell me more about that." You can also look for ways to increase change talk. We'll talk about that next.

Ways to Increase Change Talk

The acronym OARS is a good tool to help practitioners remember how to increase the occurrence of change talk.

OARS

O: Open-ended questions

A: Affirmations

R: Reflections

S: Summarizing

Open-Ended Questions

Open-ended questions allow for a conversational style to develop between provider and patient. Close questions can be answered with one-word responses—yes or no. They don't promote a real back and forth between people. Learning to phrase questions that allow for the patient to expand is an essential tool for helping the provider understand the internal goals and desires of the patient that will help them be able to foster change. Look at the questions in Table 4.1 and think about which questions would be most effective to help the provider learn about their patient.

Table 4.1 Closed verses Open Ended Questions

Closed Questions	Open-Ended Version
"Do you want to quit smoking?"	What are your thoughts about quitting smoking?"
"Is exercising important to you?"	"How does exercising fit into your life right now?"
"Is it hard for you to make healthy food choices?"	"What challenges have you experienced when trying to make healthy food choices?"
"Do you value your health?"	"What does being healthy mean to you?"
"Will you start exercising this week?"	"What might be the first step for you if you decided to start exercising?
"Have you tried to quit drinking before?"	"What have you tried in the past when you thought about quitting drinking, and how did it go?"

Affirmations

Affirmations in MI are statements that allow the provider to recognize and validate the efforts, strengths, and intentions of the patient. They help the provider to build rapport with the patient and help the patient feel understood and empowered. When done well, an affirmation can also increase self-efficacy by helping the patient feel seen and sense confidence in their abilities. For an affirmation to be used effectively, providers should follow these guidelines:

- Only offer affirmations that are sincere and reflect true observations about the patient. Affirmations are not to be used to offer generic praise or to placate the patient.
- Be specific. Offer affirmations that focus on one particular strength, effort, or quality that you observe in your patient.
- Focus on strengths. Choose an affirmation that highlights the person's abilities or their resilience in the face of their situation.
- Focus on the person when offering an affirmation, not merely on their actions, or lack thereof.

Here are some examples:

- "You've already made progress by coming in for your appointment today. That's an important first step."
- "This has been a really tough situation, and one thing I've noticed is that you've never given up. That says a lot about your sense of determination."
- "Even thinking about change is important, and you are doing that now."
- "You're really good at keeping sight of what's important to you, and that's admirable."
- "You might not have fully reached your goal, but you've put a lot of effort into making the changes that you have made, and that is worth recognizing."

Reflections

Reflective listening involves being present to take in the message that the patient is sharing with you and then being able to paraphrase what they have said to help convey to them that you understand, empathize, and want to know more. Reflections can be used to convey understanding, build rapport and collaboration, and convey feeling. When using reflections, it is important to choose your language carefully. You don't want to sound too definitive in your phrasing because you want to allow the patient to correct you and acknowledge their autonomy in this process. Using statements like "What I hear you saying is …" or "It sounds like …" can be great ways to convey this to your patient.

Reflections are not just parroting back what you've heard the patient say. They allow the patient to hear their own thoughts and emotions reflected back to them, which allows them to process and evaluate their thoughts in a different way. Doing this can help them have new insights and to lean more into change. Reflections encourage the patient to explore their thoughts and reflect on their goals and values. Reflections reduce resistance and convey a sense of nonjudgment, and they evoke change talk.

Here are some examples:

- Simple reflection to convey understanding and empathy.

  Patient: "I don't think I have time to exercise."

  Provider: "You're feeling like your schedule is already too full."

- Amplified reflection. By slightly amplifying the statement made by the patient in your reflection, you allow for the patient to reflect on the statement and perhaps consider alternatives in their thinking.

  Patient: "I don't have time to exercise."

  Provider: "It sounds like you have absolutely no time to fit exercise into your life right now."

- Reflection of feeling. This allows the provider to connect with the patient and validate their feelings.

  Patient: "It's been really hard for me to stop smoking."

  Provider: "It sounds like you are feeling frustrated and a bit overwhelmed by how difficult this change has been."

- Reflection on ambivalent statement expressed by the patient. This allows the provider to encourage the patient to explore these dualities in feeling further.

  Patient: "I enjoy drinking, but I know it's starting to cause problems in my life."

  Provider: "You like drinking because it helps you feel more relaxed, but you also see that it is getting in the way of some of your relationships."

Summarizing

Summaries draw together key points from throughout the patient's conversation. While reflections are used moment to moment, summaries pull together the big picture that the patient has been sharing, which may include things that they have shared during previous visits. Summarizing pulls together and reinforces key themes and ensures a shared understanding between patient and provider, which can help prepare the patient to decide upon next steps. Here are some tips for learning how to summarize effectively:

- Use a transition statement to draw attention to your summary and help the patient prepare to listen: "Let me summarize what I've heard so far" or "Here's what I'm understanding from our conversation."
- Draw together the most important aspects of what the patient has shared with you, including statements about change talk and feelings of ambivalence, and highlight any strengths that the patient has shared.
- Use the patient's own words whenever possible to help the summary come across as personal and authentic.
- Remember to point out any positive steps or efforts that the patient has made.
- Keep it short. Try not to overwhelm the patient by sharing back every detail. Highlight the main points to have the most clarity and impact.
- Check for accuracy. Invite the patient to confirm, clarify, or add to your summary: "Did I get that right?" or "Is there anything I missed?"
- Invite. As you close your summary, invite the patient to discuss next steps. This creates a collaborative environment, respects autonomy, and empow-

ers them to be in charge: "What are your thoughts about all that we've talked about today?" or "Where do you think we should go from here?"

KEY POINTS

- Familiarity with the process of change, including the transtheoretical model, is essential for guiding patients through transitions and addressing resistance.
- Ambivalence is a normal part of the change process; learning to work with it rather than against it is critical to effective support.
- MI offers a patient-centered framework for fostering conversations about change.
- Understanding the history and development of MI helps providers appreciate its practical and collaborative roots.
- Embodying the spirit of MI is characterized by empathy, collaboration, and respect for autonomy, which is fundamental to successful practice and facilitating change

QUESTIONS FOR REFLECTION

- Reflect on a time when you experienced significant change. How did your thoughts, feelings, and behaviors shift throughout that process?
- How does understanding the process of change help you support patients who feel stuck or resistant?
- How might identifying a patient's stage of change shape your approach to working with them?
- How could adopting the spirit of MI influence the way you interact with patients?
- Why is it important to balance guiding patients toward change while still respecting their autonomy?

SUGGESTED ACTIVITIES

1. Role-play scenario. Students pair up to practice provider-patient interactions. Providers focus on active listening, empathy, and MI techniques to identify the patient's stage of change and address ambivalence. Then, the class debriefs to discuss successes and problem solve challenges.
2. Group discussion on the following topics:
    - Challenges in identifying processes of change and strategies to overcome them

- How recognizing a patient's stage of change enhances care effectiveness
- Comparing the spirit of MI to more traditional provider-patient approaches
- Reflection on how learning this material may shift approaches to patient care
- Small-group brainstorm on how ambivalence shows up across stages and MI-based strategies to address it

3. Case study analysis. Students review (or design) case studies of patients navigating change and identify the stage of change, potential ambivalence, and MI strategies to support progress.
4. Reflective journal. Write about a time you felt ambivalent about change. What held you back? What helped you move forward? Reflect on qualities of the spirit of MI. Which do you embody most strongly, and which need further growth?

References

Derksen, F., Bensing, J. & Lagro-Janssen, A. (2013). Effectiveness of empathy in general practice: A systematic review. *British Journal of General Practice, 63*(606), e76–e84. https://doi.org/10.3399/bjgp13X660814

Dixon, L., Berger, C., & Smalley, B. (2023). The sacred space: Using stages of change model with motivational interviewing to promote patient-centered healing. *Journal of the American Psychiatric Nurses Association, 30*(3), 697–700. https://doi.org/10.1177/10783903231154607

Miller, W. R., & Rollnick, S. (2002). *Motivational interviewing: Preparing people for change* (2nd ed.). Guilford Press.

Miller, W. R., & Rollnick, S. (2023). *Motivational interviewing: Helping people change and grow* (4th ed.). Guilford Press.

Prochaska, J. O., & DiClemente, C. C. (1983). Stages and processes of self-change of smoking: Toward an integrative model of change. *Journal of Consulting and Clinical Psychology, 51*(3), 390–395. https://doi.org/10.1037/0022-006X.51.3.390

Rollnick, S., Miller, W. R., & Butler, C.C. (2008). *Motivational interviewing in healthcare: Helping patients change behavior.* Guilford Press.

Surchat, C., Carrard, V., Gaume, J., Berney, A., & Clair, C. (2022). Impact of physician empathy on patient outcomes: A gender analysis. *British Journal of General Practice, 72*(715), e99–e107. https://doi.org/10.3399/BJGP.2021.0193

Figure Credit

Fig. 4.2: William R. Miller and Stephen Rollnick, *Motivational Interviewing: Helping People Change and Grow*. Copyright © 2023 by Guilford Press.

Chapter 5

Blending MI with Other Humanistic Approaches

We think we listen, but very rarely do we listen with real understanding, true empathy. Yet listening of this very special kind, is one of the most potent forces for change that I know.

—Carl Rogers

OBJECTIVES

- Students will gain an overview of humanistic theory.
- Students will be introduced to the harm reduction model.
- Students will lean ways to collaborate with mental health providers

KEY TERMS AND DEFINITIONS

- **Congruence (genuineness)**: Being authentic and transparent in interactions with patients while maintaining professionalism.
- **Empathy**: Deeply understanding a patient's perspective without imposing personal beliefs.
- **Harm reduction**: A nonpunitive, pragmatic approach that meets patients where they are, focusing on reducing harm rather than enforcing strict compliance.
- **Unconditional positive regard (UPR)**: Accepting patients without judgment, regardless of their choices or behaviors.

The journey of psychiatry and psychology has reflected humanity's evolving understanding of mental health. In ancient times, mental illness was often attributed to supernatural or spiritual causes. People who had unusual or different behaviors were often accused of witchcraft, demonic possession, or divine punishment (Russell, 1937). This placed a sense of blame and shame on the individual or even upon their family, and treatments at the time often included harsh interventions such as rituals or exorcisms. Societies lacked the scientific structure and understanding to help them adequately contextualize and understand the complexities of human behavior. It was around the time of the Enlightenment, toward the end of the 17th century, when we saw this begin to change (Russell, 1937). The Enlightenment was a pivotal point when thinkers began to look more toward scientific inquiry than religious explanations. Still, while we began to understand that mental illness was not the result of demonic possession but instead was more connected to biological causes, our treatment for those who struggled with mental illness was highly lacking to say the least. Those considered mentally ill were shuttered away from society and housed in asylums, which lacked the basic needs for human survival such as adequate food, clothing, and access to hygiene. The mental hygiene movement began in the late 19th century and continued well into the 20th. The first seeds of the field of psychiatry emerged during this time, and we began to look at the brain and examine how neural structures influence cognitive functions, decision-making, and overall human behavior. Treatments moved toward more systematic, although still rudimentary, approaches.

This evolution continued until the late 19th and early 20th centuries, when Sigmund Freud outlined a new approach to mental health care with the introduction of his theory—psychoanalysis. Psychoanalysis put forth the idea that unconscious drives (id, ego, and superego), early childhood experiences, and repressed emotions are what shapes mental health. Freud viewed humans as driven by unconscious needs for power, aggression, and sex. He saw humans as acting in ways to meet their own needs. Freud's analytical approach emphasized the therapist as the expert who would help patients uncover their unconscious desires using techniques like free association and dream analysis. While groundbreaking, it often viewed patients in a somewhat deterministic framework, and it placed the therapist in the role of interpreter. The patient's role was to talk. Psychotherapy began to be viewed as the "talking cure."

The term "talking cure" describes how the act of talking often produced an alleviation of mental distress, also known as catharsis, through the act of verbal expression during therapy. The "talking cure" concept was popularized because of Freud and Josef Breuer's work with the famous patient, "Anna O," whose real name was Bertha Pappenheim. Anna was experiencing a wide range of physical and psychological symptoms at the time that included things like paralysis, hallucinations, and speech disturbances that could not be explained by any medical cause. Breuer found that when Anna talked about her thoughts, memories, emotions, and past traumas that her symptoms would temporarily improve. Anna coined the term "talking cure" herself (Kaplan, 2004), and it caught on.

Psychoanalysis has declined in popularity over the years for many reasons, including lack of empirical evidence, the treatment approach tends to be lengthy and costly, changing views in society that rejected some of Freud's beliefs about gender roles, culture, and sexuality (e.g., Oedipal complex), advances in neuroscience and pharmacology that focused on more biological causes and treatments for mental illness rather than unconscious drives, and changes from within psychology that made room for other approaches. However, this idea that talking can alleviate feelings of distress has remained the foundation of nearly all therapeutic approaches today.

Two approaches that developed after psychoanalysis are the behavioral and cognitive psychotherapy and humanistic psychology. Early behaviorist theories like those developed by John B. Watson and B. F. Skinner prioritize identifying and targeting observable and measurable behaviors, while cognitive approaches like those of Aaron Beck and Albert Ellis tend to address thought patterns and beliefs. One modern approach that blends behavioral and cognitive ideologies is cognitive behavioral therapy (CBT). While some may think that MI fits under the CBT category, Miller and Rollnick (2024) assert that it is a humanistic approach.

Humanistic psychology was founded by pioneers like Carl Rogers and Abraham Maslow. Their approaches emphasized a more optimistic, person-centered perspective that focused on an individual's ability for growth and change, self-actualization, and personal choice. Carl Rogers (1902–1987) is widely credited as the founder of person-centered psychotherapy. He published his first book in 1942, *Counseling and Psychotherapy*, and the approach that he introduced left an enduring mark on the field of psychotherapy. A 2006 survey conducted by Psychotherapy Networker (2007) named Rogers as the single most influential psychotherapist of the past quarter century. Rogers didn't jump on the scene with bold new techniques; rather, he led with a quiet confidence in his patients, showing practitioners that they didn't need to rely as much on set techniques but embody certain characteristics and qualities that would allow the patient to do the growth. Rogers felt strongly that the patient was the expert. Therapists served as more of a mirror. This approach serves as the foundation for the model we propose for patient-provider interactions, incorporating MI.

Rogers believed that the therapist's role was to create a space and embody certain qualities for healing to happen. He felt that the patient already had all that they needed within them to get where they needed to be. The therapist's role is to see them in a way that conveys acceptance, nonjudgment, and a positive belief in their ability to heal. He believed in the power of the therapeutic relationship as the vehicle for healing. In his 1961 book, *On Becoming a Person: A Therapist's View of Psychotherapy*, Rogers speaks of the helping relationship. He offers the following definition: "a helping relationship might be defined as one in which one of the participants intends that there should come about, in one or both parties, more appreciation of, more expression of, more functional use of the latent inner resources of the individual" (Rogers, 1961, p. 40). Rogers (1961) believed that people have internal resources they have not tapped into or that have become dormant. He felt that we could experience helping relationships in many different contexts, and he mentions the relationship between physician and patient as one of them. Rogers introduced the core characteristics of a helping relationship, and these have become the core qualities that therapists embrace when working with patients: **unconditional positive regard (UPR)**, **empathy**, and **congruence (genuineness)**. We feel that the same qualities should be present in patient-provider interactions. The relationship between provider and patient must be there in order for healing to take place, and embodying these same qualities that Rogers teaches can help this to happen in the medical setting.

Unconditional Positive Regard

Rogers defined *unconditional positive regard* as a way of accepting a person just as they are without judgment or conditions. Rogers speaks of the importance of accepting the person at all times, not just when they are behaving in ways that we deem as positive, then judging them when they are behaving in a way that we view negatively. We must reserve all judgment and offer our clients a positive feeling of approval without conditions (Rogers, 1961). When the therapist can offer a person this, it creates a safe space where they can share freely and where personal growth can be supported. Here are some examples of UPR in various contexts. Reflect on these and how it would feel to be met with UPR in these situations versus the alternative. How does being met with UPR support patient care?

In therapy:

- A person struggling with self-worth can feel free to share their feelings because their therapist conveys that they accept them just as they are.
- A person dealing with addiction feels safe, accepted, and understood rather than shamed, increasing their motivation to share feelings and work together.

In parenting:

- A child who makes mistakes (e.g., breaks a window while playing baseball in the backyard) feels supported and understood rather than shamed.
- A teenager exploring their identity feels loved and accepted by their parents.

In romantic relationships:

- A partner who feels insecure in their relationship due to a history of negative past experiences receives understanding and support instead of criticism, leading to greater emotional intimacy.
- A couple navigating conflicts learns to listen and accept each other's perspectives without conditions or judgment.

Think about your life and times when you have been met with UPR versus times when you may have been met with judgment or shame. Apply this to the medical setting and patient interactions. How might you act in ways that convey judgment? How might you change this and show UPR to your patients? What is your first thought when you encounter a patient who has lung cancer and continues to smoke? When they come back in for their checkup and are still smoking, what message do you convey? We must think about our verbal cues and our nonverbals too. Are we giving judgmental or disappointed looks? Are we using closed body language? Is what we are saying conveying a negative view on our patient?

For example, Cynthia is a patient you have been treating for diabetes. You've asked her to come in every few months to measure progress and adjust medications as needed, but she missed her last two appointments.

> *Cynthia*: "I know I should have come in sooner, but I was scared of what the test results might say."
>
> *Provider* (*who demonstrates UPR*): "I completely understand that this can be overwhelming. I'm really glad that you are here now."
>
> *Provider* (*who does not demonstrate UPR*): "Well, waiting this long didn't help. You should have come in at your appointment time. It doesn't sound like you are serious about making changes."

Which type of provider do you want to be? Which type of provider do you see yourself as?

Empathy

Empathy, or as Rogers called it, empathic understanding, is defined as the ability to deeply understand another's person's perspective, *from their perspective*, rather than imposing one's own beliefs onto the situation (Rogers, 1961). Rogers felt that empathy was a critical component of human connection, and he believed that when patients felt empathy from their therapist that therapeutic rapport could be strengthened and healing would take place. In his book *A Way of Being*, Rogers (1980) described empathy as the ability "to sense the client's private world as if it were your own, but without ever losing the 'as if' quality."

To Rogers, this meant that when the therapist feels empathy, they fully enter the patient's world, but they do not allow themselves to become overwhelmed by it. They must maintain enough therapeutic distance that they don't become completely swept away in emotion, allowing them enough space to keep the patient as the focus and to provide them with support. To express empathy adequately you must first gain an understanding of the other person's experience. This means that you must remain present and truly listen, allowing you to accurately perceive a person's emotions and experiences. You must also remain nonjudgmental, accepting that person's perception without trying to alter, judge, or criticize it. Rogers (1961) spoke of how rare it is for us to experience true empathy. He mentions that we often express empathy in the following way: I understand what you have been through. I have been through it myself, and I handled it very differently than you. This type of communication conveys an external lens and one of comparison and judgment. To Rogers, empathy is suspending analysis and judgment and conveying connection with what that person is experiencing in the moment. Rogers (1961) felt that if we could do this then the patient could "blossom and grow" (p. 62). He felt that if we were able to achieve this level of understanding and separation from our own experiences and judgment we must communicate this to the patient. They need to know that we do understand, so making statements that reflect to them that we have heard their message and are with them in this moment are key. Examples of empathic statements in health care include the following:

Example 1:

Patient: "I've been dealing with this pain for years, and no one seems to care or understand how much it impacts my life."

Provider: "That sounds incredibly frustrating and exhausting. It must be really hard to feel unheard and misunderstood. I assure you that I am listening, and I do see what you are going through."

Example 2:

Patient: "I don't have a problem! I don't know why you keep saying that I do. I'm fine. I just need medication for my pain. I am not a junkie!"

Provider: "I hear you. It sounds like you are really frustrated because you feel that I am making assumptions about you. That is really difficult. My job isn't to label you. I want to work with you to understand your experience and see how I can support you in a way that makes sense for you and what we are dealing with here."

In this second example, we see an instance when the patient is frustrated with the provider and may even have an escalated tone or animated nonverbals We've all been in these situations. It can be very easy to become defensive in these instances. However, often learning to depersonalize what the patient is saying and viewing it as not an attack on you, but a reaction out of fear, frustration, or other emotions in relation to what they are going through is the most helpful scenario. If that example were to play out the patient would likely still not receive the medication that they are asking for, but perhaps some compromises can take place along the way. Perhaps displaying and feeling empathy for our patients will help us to create a strong working connection with them so that we can find some way to work together. In many alternatives, the patient merely leaves angry, without their medication, to either try something else or perhaps seek out other, less safe methods for self-medication. Empathy is not a blanket that washes over the provider's ability to hold true when it comes to medical expertise, but it can be a bridge that allows patients to continue to feel safe and supported so that they want to come in and work toward healthier solutions.

Congruence

The third of the core conditions of effective therapeutic relationships that Rogers identified is congruence, also known as genuineness. Rogers viewed this to mean that the therapist is demonstrating authenticity in the session instead of presenting a false front or facade. He was basically saying to be true to who you are. Instead of putting on a clinical mask, be open and honest with your emotions. Be consistent in feelings, words, and actions. Demonstrate integrity. Do what you say that you will do. If you say you will follow up on providing a resource to a patient, do it. Respect their time, boundaries, and rights as a person. There is also an element of emotional presence within the condition of congruence. Be present and engaged with the patient. Don't be distracted, detached, or distant. This might be challenging for providers who tend to look at their computer screen more than the patient. Making a small shift, to turn to face the patient instead of the computer screen, could go a long way to connect with them. In his 1961 book *On Becoming a Person*, Rogers explains the concept of congruence as the therapist is "openly being the feelings and attitudes which at that moment are flowing *in* him" (p. 61). In other words, you do not have to hide or pretend that you are not feeling what you feel with your patients. You are genuine and authentic. You acknowledge what you feel, and if appropriate you share them. Think of your interactions with people. You can tell when they mean what they say versus when they don't. Authenticity matters, and when it is present patients can feel it. When it is not, patients can feel that too. An example that Rogers (1961) gives is to think of the put-off feeling that we have when we hear TV personalities speak at times; it is often due to feeling like they are putting on an act and not being "real."

In addition to my work as a counselor, educator, and therapist, I am also a yoga instructor. When I completed my 200-hour yoga teacher training we talked a bit about being careful to be the same person in the yoga room as I am in the lobby greeting students. My yoga mentor said to watch for slipping into a "yoga voice." She meant that I don't need to lose all sense of humanity and connection and slip into some kind of guru-like personality that doesn't connect with who I am. Sure, I might speak more slowly or offer cues and instructions in a calmer pace, but I can still convey a sense of who I am. You don't drop that away the moment you walk in to begin the class. There are different versions of ourselves that are still genuine to who we are in different situations. The version of me that you might see at a concert might look a bit different than the version you'd see in the grocery store, but all connection between the two situations is not lost. The same basic person underlies each of these scenarios.

One might wonder how providers can display congruence while also maintaining professionalism. It is important to note that congruence in therapeutic or professional settings means that the person is authentic and open. It does not mean that they share every thought and feeling that comes into their minds in an impulsive or judgmental way. Rather, a skilled practitioner who embodies this quality can find balance among honesty, professionalism, and nonjudgmental acceptance. They can make sure that the demonstration of their own feelings and reactions supports the client's growth rather than impose their own reactions and values onto the patient. Providers must learn to monitor their own thoughts and reactions and choose when and how to express them. We should always ask ourselves if we are acting in a way that benefits our clients. For example, instead of reacting to a patient who is resisting change with frustration, the provider acknowledges this internal feeling and then reframes their response into something constructive. Some questions providers might ask themselves when learning to practice congruence include these:

- Is what I am about to say supportive of the patient's growth?
- Am I responding from a place of personal reactivity?
- Am I bringing a sense of emotional presence without blurring professional boundaries?

These are great questions to consider because they help us become aware of internal reaction patterns. If we find ourselves wanting to say something, but we find that it is not supportive of the patient's growth, that is something we can notice, reflect on, and find a way to balance truthfulness and constructive feedback in our communication. Simple changes in phrasing can help us here. Instead of saying "Your weight has not changed," a provider could say, "I notice you are struggling to make changes in your life; can we talk about why that might be?"

If we find that we respond from a sense of personal reactivity, this reflects our own situations, not the patient's. When this happens, it is important to consider a concept in psychology called transference, which was described by Sigmund Freud. Transference is when someone projects their own thoughts, feelings, and reactions onto someone else based on our own past experiences (Szasz, 1963). This can happen when working with patients. Maybe we had an alcoholic parent ourselves, and we have a patient who is struggling with alcoholism or another behavior that reminds us of that parent that we saw as unwilling to change. These reactions are not always on the surface. Transference often happens unconsciously, but when we learn to slow down and monitor our reactions, we can become more aware and able to slow down our reactions to it. We can learn to reflect and pause, and instead of reacting with frustration or judgment, we can reframe our response in a way that focuses on acknowledging our patient's feelings and working together to come up with a solution. For example, instead of responding to a patient that we view as stubborn and unwilling to engage in help and saying "You don't seem to want to listen to what I am telling you to do," we could say, "I can tell this is a challenge for you, and the ideas that I am sharing do not seem like they will work for you. Can we talk about why that is and work together to find something that might benefit you?" The term "transference" is used when the patient projects their feelings onto the provider, and the term "countertransference" is used when the provider experiences this projection toward the patient. Both things can take place, and while this may be viewed as problematic, when we learn to monitor for transference (maybe my patient seems overly upset with me due to something other than just me) and countertransference (am I overly reacting to my patient?), we can gain a lot of information that can help us form a deeper working relationship. It is all about how we respond when we notice that transference is taking place. Recognizing and reframing our reaction is a huge piece of the puzzle.

To ensure that we are balancing emotional presence with professional boundaries, it is important to relate without oversharing. In therapy, we talk a lot about the appropriateness of self-disclosure. There can be appropriate times to self-disclose, but we must first ask ourselves if the self-disclosure is helping our patient or if we are making the discussion about us instead of about them. Another thing to watch for is offering emotional support without making promises that we cannot keep. Our patients often experience huge challenges, and while we do want to be there for them and relate, we don't want to guarantee a certain outcome that we cannot follow through on. This is when we can offer guidance, share our expertise, and empower our patients to make their own decisions. When we don't know for certain, it is okay to share that with empathy and presence. Instead of saying, "Oh, I know you'll be okay," you might try saying, "I can't predict exactly what will happen here, but I can promise to do everything possible to help you through it. You are not alone."

Rogers's ideas shifted the focus from diagnosing and treating mental illness to understanding the person as a whole, which includes understanding their strengths, aspirations, and lived experiences. Many modern approaches evolved from the teachings of Rogers, including MI (Miller & Rollnick, 2024). Much like the theory of Rogers, Miller and Rollnick (2024) do not view MI as a collection of behavioral techniques and gimmicks but as an approach or way of being. They have always described MI by calling it the "spirit of MI." Rogers, likewise, called his approach "attitudes" or key concepts. We don't just put our empathy hats on. We are people who show empathy. It is who we are.

I often tell my counseling students that who *they are* is the tool for change. For the most part, counselors don't use a tool outside of themselves, such as a saw, hammer, or computer to "get a job done." Certainly, there are biofeedback tools, tappers, or other instruments that a counselor may use when working with a client. We collaborate with medical professionals who may run bloodwork or other assessments that provide useful information, and there are a wide array of clinical assessments that we may administer to help us gain insight into a person's functioning, but so much of what we do with a person is interpersonal, and how we present to them and the level with which we are able to show up is the tool. *We are the tool.* Who we are and the qualities that we embody are the tools for change. The more we improve and work on ourselves, and the more we understand and embody our chosen therapeutic orientation, the better we will be able to be present for them. As medical providers there are certainly tools that are used in practice, but much of the same concept is true for patient interactions as well. Who you are as a person and how you interact with your patients will make the biggest difference.

One quality that Rollnick and Miller (2024) added to MI beyond Rogers's three core concepts of unconditional positive regard, empathy, and congruence is the quality of empowerment. The patient is empowered to make decisions and to lead their journey forward. We convey this to them through our collaborative work together. We provide guidance on the path, as experts with knowledge, but they decide which way to go. They lead the way. Rogers's core concepts brought essential humanistic qualities to the table that serve as tools to create an environment for clients to change. MI does this as well but expands on it by actively empowering people through the spirit of the approach, which adds a more direct element of empowerment than Rogers developed with his person-centered theory.

Maslow

Another key contributor to humanistic psychology worth noting is Abraham Maslow. His most widely known contribution was his hierarchy of needs, which was presented briefly in Chapter 3. Maslow's hierarchy of needs is connected to his ideas surrounding human potential and growth toward a concept called *self-actualization*. Maslow (1958) viewed self-actualization as the best version of ourselves. By pointing out that humans have basic survival needs (food, water, shelter), safety needs (security, stability, health, financial security), needs for love and belonging (relationships, friendships, intimacy, community), and esteem needs (a need for recognition, self-worth, accomplishment) that are essential for us to have met in order to attain self-actualization, Maslow shifted the focus within the field of psychology from only examining dysfunction within individuals to exploring well-being, potential, and motivation. How can we help people to meet their needs so that they can become their best selves? Maslow shifted the focus in ways that made society as a whole look at how we help each other on this journey toward self-actualization. We started examining society to understand how accessible or challenging it is for different groups to have their needs met within the existing social structure. It has created the need for deep reflection on the factors that make it harder for some people to get ahead compared to others. Racism, sexism, ableism, and a whole host of other factors are real barriers for many in our society, and this is an important concept to remember with our patients when they come in. How are they doing on the need's hierarchy? Are there areas that we can identify and resources that we can provide to help them better meet or address various aspects of their live?

Here are some questions to consider when talking with patients that could help you to understand how well their needs are being met:

Physiological needs (basic survival)

- Do you have access to food and clean drinking water?
- Have you been experiencing any issues related to sleeping?
- Do you have access to everything that you need to take care of personal hygiene?

Safety needs (security and stability)

- Do you feel safe where you live?
- Do you have any fears related to your housing situation in the near future?
- Do you have any concerns about your own safety or that of your family?
- Do you have stable employment or a source of income to meet your basic needs?

Love and belonging (social support and relationships)

- Do you have close friends or family members that you can turn to for support?
- Do you feel isolated or lonely?
- Do you have connections that help you feel loved and valued?

Esteem needs (self-worth and confidence)

- Have you been able to engage in activities that give you a sense of purpose?
- Are there any goals or personal achievements that you are working toward?
- Do you struggle with feelings of self-doubt or low confidence?

Self-actualization (personal growth and fulfillment)

- Are you able to pursue activities or interests that bring you joy?
- Do you feel like you are living in alignment with your values and beliefs?
- What motivates you and gives your life meaning?

These can be great questions to help you understand your patient—what they need help with and what they hope to experience in life. We might be able to help connect them with community resources to help offer support for some of the basic needs of life, and inquiring about their personal values, goals, and desires can help us to know how we can support them in these efforts. Often what we think a patient needs is different from what they feel that they need. Take interest and allow them to educate you in this area. It is one way to support the whole person.

As a mental health professional, studying this field fascinates me, and wanting to help find and improve approaches to mental health treatment has been one of my most driving forces. I find myself eager to share what I know. I am also very motivated to collaborate from an interdisciplinary lens because I hope that in doing so, we can elevate how mental health is viewed in society, in general. There tends to be stigmatization when it comes to mental health treatments in comparison to physical health. If someone breaks a bone, we tell them that they need to see a doctor, have an X-ray, get a cast. There is rarely shame or judgment. However, when someone struggles with depression so debilitating that they cannot leave their home, they are often met with statements like these:

- "Snap out of it."
- "Try harder."
- "Think happy thoughts."
- "Have you thought about eating healthier?"
- "You should just try to exercise."

This needs to change, and one of the main reasons for working to spread the message discussed in this text is an effort to collaborate with nurses, doctors, and all medical professionals so that we can see the value of working together across disciplines and learn from one another. Primary care providers see patients who are trapped in negative cycles, unable to move forward due to unhealthy thinking patterns or habits that keep them stuck. They also see patients struggling with addiction, depression, diabetes, and other health conditions that require them to learn to think differently. For years medical professionals have prescribed solutions and wondered why patients didn't follow through, which has led to widespread provider burnout, as witnessed over the past 10 years, at a time when we need all hands on deck.

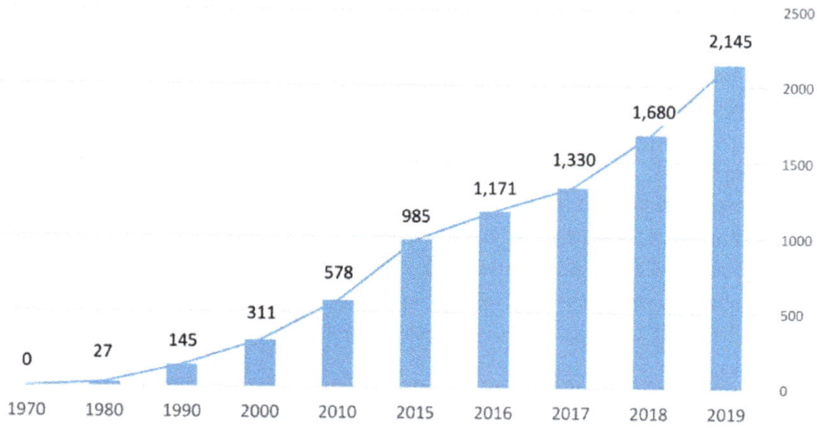

Figure 5.1 Provider Burnout Rates (De Hert, 2020)

When I began my entry into the world of mental health as a young provisionally licensed counselor, I attended a training on MI. At that training, the leader shared a story that has always stuck with me. She said that when she began working in community support, she had a client who was unhoused. He was living in a tent; he had advanced cancer, multiple mental health diagnoses, limited food resources, and almost no family support. When she began developing goals for him, she created a list. First, get him housing. Second, get him treatment for his cancer. Third, work on medication compliance for his depression. Fourth, create a support network for him. She began her interactions with him with these preestablished goals in mind, and she found that it was not working. He was not engaged during their appointments. He didn't follow through with any of the ideas that she had for him. He just lived his life and sort of tolerated her when she came by for her appointments. Finally, one day out of desperation she asked him what he wanted, and he said, "I'd like to get a fishing pole and go fishing more." She was floored. Was this really all that he felt he needed, even with all that he had going on? She didn't know how to respond, but as she sat with it more, she saw that this was how he wanted to spend the rest of his life. His cancer diagnosis was terminal. She couldn't change that or have him committed to a facility. He was not a danger to himself, and he was competent to make decisions. She finally realized that this man had the right to spend the rest of his days living in a tent if he wanted, and if his quality of life would be improved by fishing, then she could help him with that. She switched her lens and began to see that if she chose to honor and support this goal with him first, maybe they could work on other things later, and if not, at least he had something that held meaning added back into his days. She learned that if she could help him get a fishing pole so he could go fishing, she *did* actually improve his quality of life. Maybe he viewed life and prioritized his situation differently, and as hard as that was for her, she saw that these were his decisions to make. Once she helped him to achieve that goal, she was able to establish trust and then continue to work with him to not fully change his situation to the point that she was happy with where he was, but his goals were first, and she was able to make headway to help him make improvements that benefitted his safety. He became willing to make small changes, agreeing to use a bus in the community to show up for his treatments, for example.

Looking at patient interactions in this way requires a real mindset shift, and we get that this takes time, but once we make that shift, we can see that we never really controlled the outcome through merely prescribing solutions anyway. The patient always has. They need to follow through, and when we let them teach us enough to allow us to know how to best help and support them, we see the best outcomes.

Reframing Change Through a Harm Reduction Lens

Another important theory to add to our discussion is that of **harm reduction**. Harm Reduction International (n.d.b.) defines *harm reduction* as "policies, programs and practices that aim to minimise the negative health, social, and legal impacts associated with drug use, drug policies, and drug laws" (para. 1). They further elaborate that harm reduction is based in "justice and human rights. It focuses on positive change and on working with people without judgement, coercion, discrimination, or requiring that people stop using drugs as a precondition of support" (para. 2).

The harm reduction movement started in the 1970s and 1980s in response to the growing public health concerns related to substance use, particularly heroin injection and the spread of the HIV/AIDS epidemic. It was a grassroots movement that aimed to provide support through pragmatic rather than punitive approaches. Dr. Russell Newcombe is credited with coining the term "harm reduction" in his 1987 article "High Time for Harm Reduction."

Some of the strategies that we have seen evolve out of the harm reduction lens are things like needle exchange programs, which became popular in the Netherlands and the United Kingdom. These programs aim to reduce the risk of spreading diseases like hepatitis and HIV that are associated with injection drug use. We have also seen promotion of safe injection sites (SISs), also known as supervised consumption site (SCSs); individuals can use substances that they have previously obtained under the supervision of trained medical staff. Staff at these sites can provide sterile needles, supervise consumption, and respond immediately, if needed, by administering medications like naloxone (Narcan). Currently 93 countries offer needle and syringe programs, 94 offer opioid agonist therapy, 18 countries have drug consumption rooms, and 108 countries support harm reduction in their national policies (Harm Reduction International, n.d.a.). The United States opened its first government-sanctioned SIS in 2021 in

New York City but continues to have very few sites in comparison to other countries.

Other harm reduction approaches that have had more success gaining traction are things like the decriminalization of marijuana and other substances, methadone maintenance therapy, and public education on safer drug use and overdose prevention. Another harm reduction ideology that has caught on is the Good Samaritan Law, which allows people to call for medical help during a drug overdose, even if illegal drugs are present at the scene, without fear of legal consequences (Schneider et al., 2022). As of May 2024, 48 states and the District of Columbia have fatal overdose prevention laws under Good Samaritan; only Kansas and Wyoming do not (Legislative Analysis and Public Policy Association, 2024). The idea is that we want to encourage people to seek emergency assistance without fear of arrest. The entire harm reduction philosophy is to provide help and support for those who need it instead of punitive actions that might force someone to continue to act in ways that are unhealthy or dangerous.

Gabor Maté (2010), a Canadian physician and author of *In the Realm of Hungry Ghosts: Close Encounters With Addiction*, says the following about harm reduction:

> Harm reduction is often perceived as being inimical to the ultimate purpose of "curing" addiction—that is, of helping addicts transcend their habits and heal. People regard it as "coddling" addicts, as enabling them to continue their destructive ways. It's also considered to be the opposite of abstinence, which many regard as the only legitimate goal of addiction treatment. Such a distinction is artificial. The issue in medical practice is always how best to help a patient. If a cure is possible and probable without doing greater harm, then cure is the objective. When it isn't—and in most chronic medical conditions cure is not the expected outcome—the physician's role is to help the patient with the symptoms and to reduce the harm done by the disease process. In rheumatoid arthritis, for example, one aims to prevent joint inflammation and bone destruction and, in all events, to reduce pain. In incurable cancers we aim to prolong life, if that can be achieved without a loss of life quality, and also to control symptoms. In other words, harm reduction means making the lives of afflicted human beings more bearable, more worth living. That is also the goal of harm reduction in the context of addiction.
>
> Although hardcore drug addiction is much more than a disease, the harm reduction model is essential to its treatment. Given our lack of a systematic, evidence-based approach to addiction, in many cases it's futile to dream of a cure. So long as society ostracizes the addict and the legal system does everything

> it can to heighten the drug problem, the welfare and medical systems can aim only to mitigate some of its effects. Sad to say, in our context harm reduction means reducing not only the harm caused by the disease of addiction, but also the harm caused by the social assault on drug addicts. (p. 332)

We can apply harm reduction principles in areas beyond addiction as well. For example, when treating chronic health conditions like emphysema or diabetes, we can move from an all-or-nothing lens to one of supporting positive changes and minimizing harm. For emphysema, we can change our thinking to encourage patients to cut back from smoking rather than expect that they quit immediately. We could focus on things like pulmonary rehab and light physical activity to improve lung function and suggest breathing exercises to help manage shortness of breath. For diabetes, we could view blood sugar management without the addition of shame. We could allow flexibility in carb counting instead of restrictive meal plans. We could encourage small, sustainable dietary changes, like reducing portion sizes instead of telling people to completely eliminate favorite foods. We could alter our language to avoid using terms like "bad" versus "good" blood sugar levels. A harm reduction approach to conditions like emphysema and diabetes acknowledges the lifelong nature and complexity of these illnesses. It allows us to see the overall needs of the whole person and how smoking or how certain "off-limits" foods do add an element of pleasure into people's lives. It promotes seeking balance by prioritizing small, manageable changes to improve health outcomes while understanding individual circumstances rather than shaming and demanding immediate, perfect adherence to medical prescriptions.

Gentsch et al. (2024) interviewed adults who had type 1 or type 2 diabetes to understand their relationship with food and found that the participants in their study often used language associated with addiction when they talked about food. They referred to themselves as "addicts" and described food as a "drug." The study participants also viewed times when they would indulge in unhealthy eating as "cheating" or as a personal weakness and often spoke about food's ability to provide comfort to their emotions, indicating that this was one of the factors that made it most difficult to refrain from unhealthy foods and sustain a healthy diet. The conclusion from this study was to encourage providers to consider using a harm reduction lens when working with patients who describe their relationship with food as addictive. Gentsch et al. (2024) cite the effectiveness of harm reduction approaches with other addiction populations and encourage the consideration of this model with patients who have diabetes in order to decrease shame and stigma related with diabetes and increase quality of life for patients.

Providers are Not Alone

We want to take a moment here to acknowledge that working as a medical provider is hard. The job, as is, is already an uphill battle with patient needs, insurance and billing constraints, limits on time, and trying to find a moment for self-care and work-life balance in the midst of it all. We know that it can feel impossible. We know that providers are trying their best. The ideas in this book may take time and dedication to learn. It does require a mindset shift, but in the next chapter we will show that MI has been shown to be effective, not just in patient outcomes and satisfaction but in provider satisfaction as well. The use of MI and the underlying principles of humanistic psychology have helped many providers to connect with the passion that brought them to the profession in the first place. We want these tools to help you to feel less pressure related to outcomes with patients. We want you to focus on connecting with patients, listening to them, providing your expertise, and then allowing them to decide. We hope in some ways it takes pressure off you rather than adds to it.

We also want you to know that we are calling for an increase in collaboration between medical providers and mental health professionals. These are not separate disciplines. They are overlapping branches of the same one. We, as mental health provider and medical provider, see ourselves as extensions of the same goal, which is treating the whole person. We ask that more medical offices partner with counselors, and vice versa. Collaborate, partner, and learn from and with one another. This will benefit patients in numerous ways by allowing them to see the two disciplines as less separate. We know from research that mental health and wellness impact physical health, and the same is true in reverse. Books like *The Body Keeps the Score* by Bessel van der Kolk (2014) and *When the Body Says No: Exploring the Stress Disease Connection* by Gabor Maté (2003) illustrate the connection between mind and body. Let us join in and work together as one.

In the next chapter, we will present data related to the use of techniques like MI and the impact it has on health outcomes. Specifically, we will look at how MI leads to improved patient satisfaction, enhanced clinical outcomes, and improved provider satisfaction and fulfillment. We will also look at how increasing interdisciplinary collaboration between medical and mental health providers supports more holistic patient care, increases effectiveness, and enhances outcomes for both patients and providers.

KEY POINTS

- Mental illness was historically misunderstood, often attributed to supernatural causes, leading to stigmatization and inhumane treatments. Over time, scientific understanding has shifted toward biological, psychological, and humanistic approaches.

- While Freud's psychoanalytic approach laid the foundation for talk therapy, it was later replaced by cognitive behavioral approaches and humanistic psychology, which emphasize growth, self-actualization, and a person-centered perspective.
- Rogers introduced the core conditions for therapeutic change—UPR, empathy, and congruence (genuineness)—which are essential for both mental health professionals and medical providers.
- MI, developed by Miller and Rollnick, aligns with Rogers's humanistic principles by emphasizing collaboration, patient autonomy, and empowerment rather than coercion or direct persuasion.
- Understanding where patients are on Maslow's hierarchy can help providers address unmet needs (e.g., food, housing, social support) before expecting behavioral changes.
- Instead of an all-or-nothing stance on behavior change, harm reduction supports small, realistic improvements to minimize harm, especially in chronic health conditions like diabetes, emphysema, and addiction.
- Mental and physical health are deeply connected, requiring greater collaboration between medical providers and mental health professionals for holistic patient care.
- By embodying humanistic principles, providers reduce burnout, foster deeper patient trust, and increase the likelihood of meaningful behavior change.

QUESTIONS FOR REFLECTION

- Reflect on your approach to patient care. How do you incorporate Rogers's principle of empathy, UPR, and genuineness in your interactions? Write about a time when you felt you successfully used these principles and about a time when you feel you could have improved.
- Think back on a time when you found it challenging to accept a patient's outlook, choices, or behaviors. How could you apply Rogerian principles to change this interaction?
- How might unmet needs (food insecurity, unstable housing, living in an unsafe environment, lacking social connections and supports) impact a person's ability to work toward behavior change?
- How can health care providers help patients address basic needs as they arise?
- What is your personal stance on harm reduction approaches (education about substance use, needle exchanges, supportive medications like methadone)?
- How does harm reduction challenge traditional thoughts, beliefs, and approaches that promote abstinence or complete adherence to prescribed interventions?

- What are some of the goals of harm reduction approaches? What are some of the common misconceptions?
- How can you learn from and collaborate with mental health providers to benefit your patients?

SUGGESTED ACTIVITIES

1. Create an empathy map for a patient struggling with addiction or behavior change. Divide your map into four quadrants that address the following questions:
   - What is the patient thinking?
   - What is the patient feeling?
   - What are they saying?
   - What are they doing?

   Discuss how this exercise could help you to better understand the patient's perspective of their situation and barriers to change.

2. Create a behavior change plan with your patient who is working toward smoking cessation. When designing your plan think about how you can incorporate what we have learned about humanistic psychology, MI, and harm reduction thus far.
   - Using Maslow's hierarchy, think about how to understand the patient's needs first.
   - How could you inquire about this information through use of a person-centered, MI approach?
   - How could the harm reduction lens help you work with this patient in a way that promotes growth rather than an all-or-nothing approach?
   - Reflect on how this approach is different from a strict, compliance-based medical model.

3. Many people, including providers, have strong opinions about harm reduction strategies like safe injection sites, needle exchange programs, and medication-assisted treatment for addiction. Reflect on your personal feelings about this issue Answer the following questions, either by yourself or as a group.
   - Do you believe harm reduction is effective?
   - Discuss the ethical dilemmas related to these approaches.
   - How does harm reduction align with Rogers's humanistic approach and the principles of MI?
   - Do you see any relationship between harm reduction principles and Maslow's needs hierarchy?

References

De Hert, S. (2020). Burnout in healthcare workers: Prevalence, impact, and preventative strategies. *Local and Regional Anesthesia, 13*, 171–183. https://doi.org/10.2147/lra.s240564

Gentsch, A., Reed, M., Cunningham, A., Chang, A., Kahn, S., Kovalsky, D., Doty, A., Mills, G., Hollander, J., & Rising, K. (2024, January 2). *"Once I take that one bite": The consideration of harm reduction as a strategy to support dietary change for patients with diabetes*. Jefferson Digital Commons. https://jdc.jefferson.edu/healthpolicyfaculty/189/

Harm Reduction International. (n.d.a.). *The global state of harm reduction*. https://hri.global/flagship-research/the-global-state-of-harm-reduction/

Harm Reduction International. (n.d.b.). *What is harm reduction?* https://hri.global/what-is-harm-reduction/

Kaplan. (2004). O Anna: Being Bertha Pappenheim—historiography and biography. *Australasian Psychiatry, 12*(1), 62–68. https://doi.org/10.1046/j.1039-8562.2003.02062.x

Legislative Analysis and Public Policy Association. (2024). *Good Samaritan fatal overdose prevention and drug-induced homicide: Summary of state laws*. https://legislativeanalysis.org/wp-content/uploads/2024/05/Good-Samaritan-Fatal-Overdose-Prevention-Summary-of-State-Laws.pdf

Maslow, A. H. (1958). Understanding human motivation. In C. L. Stacey & M. DeMartino (Eds.), *A dynamic theory of human motivation* (pp. 26–47). Howard Allen. https://doi.org/10.1037/11305-004

Maté, G. (2003). *When the body says no: Understanding the stress-disease connection*. John Wiley & Sons.

Maté, G. (2010). *In the realm of hungry ghosts: Close encounters with addiction*. North Atlantic Books.

Miller, W. R., & Rollnick, S. (2024). Why motivational interviewing is a person-centered approach. *Sucht, 70*(2), 97–101. https://doi.org/10.1024/0939-5911/a000862

Rogers, C. R. (1961). *On becoming a person: A therapist's view of psychotherapy*. Houghton Mifflin.

Rogers, C. R. (1980). *A way of being*. Houghton Mifflin.

Russell, W. (1937). The evolution of psychiatry. *South African Journal of Science, 34*, 121–134.

Schneider, K. E., Park, J., Allen, S. T., Weir, B. W., & Sherman, S. G. (2022). Good Samaritan laws. *Public Health Reports, 135*(3). https://doi.org/10.1177/0033354920915439

Szasz, T. S. (1963). The concept of transference. *The International Journal of Psycho-Analysis, 44*(4), 432–443.

Van der Kolk, B. A. (2014). *The body keeps the score: Brain, mind, and body in the healing of trauma*. Viking.

Figure Credit

Fig. 5.1: Stefan De Hert, "Burnout in Healthcare Workers: Prevalence, Impact and Preventative Strategies," *Local and Regional Anesthesia*, vol. 13, p. 172, https://www.dovepress.com/
burnout-in-healthcare-workers-prevalence-impact-and-preventative-strat-peer-reviewed-fulltext-article-LRA. Copyright © 2020 by Taylor & Francis Group.

Chapter 6

Integrating MI with the Nursing Process

You treat a disease: you win, you lose. You treat a person, I guarantee you win ... no matter the outcome.

—*Robin Williams,* Patch Adams

We have often heard that nursing is an art, but what exactly is that art? Hildegard Peplau (1988) described nursing as an art form that shares similarities with both the performing and visual arts, such as dance, music, painting, and sculpture. She emphasized that, like these art forms, nursing has the power to deeply move and personally impact individuals through the nurse's practice. Nurses connect to patients in some of their most vulnerable times. Listening, caring, supporting, and encouraging patients are part of the daily routine. MI skills fit perfectly with the nursing process, and we will explore more of that "art" in this chapter.

OBJECTIVES

- Students will be able to define the evolution of the nursing process.
- Students will be able to apply the core principles of MI to the nursing process.
- Students will be able to discuss how MI can be applied in real-life scenarios for nurses.
- Students will demonstrate an understanding of the benefits of MI as evidence-based practice for communication techniques.

KEY TERM AND DEFINITION

- **Clinical judgment measurement model**: Sometimes referred to as the next-generation NCLEX model; a model that was introduced by the National Council of State Boards of Nursing that emphasizes cognitive processes in clinical decision-making such as recognizing and analyzing cues, prioritizing hypotheses, generating solutions, acting, and evaluating outcomes.

The art and science of nursing is a complex interplay between evidence-based practice and patient-centered care. Nurses are often at the forefront of people's lives when they are the most vulnerable, and nurses must possess compassion, empathy, and understanding for their fellow man. Often a nurse will find a patient expresses gratitude for the care they have received, and that is their reward for working long hours, seeing patients, or catching up on notes during a lunch or bathroom break, and spending holidays and weekends away from your family. Nursing operates under a defined *scope of practice*, which outlines the services that nurses are trained, competent, and authorized to perform. These regulations are set by the Nursing Practice Act (NPA), which differs from state to state. Central to nursing practice is the *nursing process*, which we have spoken briefly about in previous chapters.

The nursing process is a systematic, organized approach to how nurses provide individualized care and initially consisted of ADPIE—assessment, diagnosis, planning, implementation, and evaluation—but this model has been revised with the next-generation NCLEX (NGN). The National Council of State Boards of Nursing (NCSBN) introduced the **clinical judgment measurement model** (NCJMM) emphasizing the cognitive processes involved in the clinical decision-making process. The thought is to train nurses on how they make clinical judgments in real-life situations to enhance their preparedness for entry into practice and involves the following stages:

1. Recognize the cues.
2. Analyze them.
3. Prioritize hypothesis.
4. Generate solutions.
5. Act.
6. Evaluate outcomes.

Both the NGN model and MI focus on patient-centered care in a slightly different but important way. The NGN model encourages nurses to take into consideration patient preferences and collaborate with them in planning. The nurse examines the cues and analyzes them, then comes up with a structured plan that takes into consideration patients' wants and needs. MI takes it one step further and focuses on exploring what a patient's personal motivations, values, and goals are to elicit a behavior change. With the NGN model the *nurse comes up with the plan* that is patient centered. With MI the plan and the motivation *come from the patient* with the nurse supporting them. Think about this small shift in perception. In the following case study, evaluate how each method makes you feel and ask yourself which one you would be more inclined to follow if you were Jessica or her mom.

Case Study

The patient is a 12-year-old girl who is on the border of obesity. The past year her family has undergone multiple changes due to the COVID-19 pandemic. She has had to attend school virtually on Zoom. To accommodate this change in schedule the parents work opposite shifts. Mom works in the evening so that she can supervise Jessica in the day, and Dad works in the daytime. Dad works in road construction and is very tired coming home, so he usually picks up fast food for him and Jessica to eat. Jessica has not been able to play much with her friends because of the COVID restrictions. She has mainly spent the last year watching school on Zoom or playing video games. But summer is coming, and school restrictions have been lifted, so things will be changing. The provider has indicated that Jessica and her family need to engage in more exercise and have a better diet. You have been assigned to work with them on making some lifestyle changes that involve more exercise for Jessica and better meals.

NGN Approach: Patient Centered

Recognize the Cues

The nurse gathers all the information, noting that Jessica has gained weight over the past year and has an elevated BMI. Jessica is currently not attending school in person, which contributes to decreased physical activity. Most of her time is spent on technology or in Zoom classes, and her diet is mainly composed of takeout or highly processed foods that she consumes with her family at home.

Analyze the Cues

The family dynamics have changed over the past year, causing lots of changes at home. Mom is working at night, which means Dad is responsible for dinner. It sounds like dad has a labor-intensive job or is not interested in cooking at home because he is grabbing take-out for Jessica. Jessica is not attending school or playing with friends due to COVID restrictions, so she is getting much less activity than she usually does.

Prioritize Hypothesis

The nurse considers the most pressing issue to be Jessica's weight gain and wants to prevent her from progressing from borderline obesity into the obesity classification. The nurse also has secondary concerns related to mental health and family stress due to the COVID-19 disruptions.

Generate Solutions

The nurse asks for suggestions from Jessica and her family about how they would like to change their eating habits or exercise and takes them into consideration when developing the care plan. The nurse educates Jessica and her family about the dangers of obesity and how a well-rounded diet is important to ward off chronic diseases like diabetes. She also discusses the current recommendations for a healthy diet from the CDC and exercise and screening recommendations. The nurse then develops a plan suggesting specific evidence-based interventions such as setting a daily schedule for physical activity, planning family meals, and reducing screen time.

Act

The nurse implements the plan by providing the family with a written schedule incorporating SMART (specific, measurable, achievable, realistic, and timely) goals. Jessica will complete a 20-minute walk every night after dinner and will incorporate three vegetables a day into her diet within the next 2 weeks.

Evaluate Outcomes

The nurse will schedule a follow-up appointment or phone call to see how the family is progressing with the cocreated goals.

Sample NGN Dialogue

> *Nurse*: "Jessica, I see that you've been doing school from home and your family's routine has changed a lot this year. I understand that it's been hard to stay active and eat healthy. Based on what your doctor recommended, I'd like to help you and your family set up a daily routine that includes some fun physical activities and healthy meals. What do you think about that?"
>
> *Jessica*: "That sounds good."
>
> *Nurse*: "Exercise is important for your growing body. What are some fun things you like to do?"
>
> *Mom*: "Yeah, we have really gotten off track."

Nurse: "It's okay, we can come up with a plan you will like."

Jessica: "I like riding my bike and taking the dog for a walk."

Nurse: "How about we start with a 20-minute walk after dinner each night?"

Jessica: "Okay."

Nurse: "Eating out every night is bad for your body. Sodas have a lot of sugar in them, and they are hard on your teeth. How about we find a way to add some fruits and vegetables to your day and make some fun meals at home?"

Mom: "My husband is not much of a cook, and he is exhausted when he gets home. Making dinners has been a real challenge."

Nurse: "There are some great apps on the CDC website that can help you plan meals easily. Why don't we take a look and see what they have?"

Mom: "Okay."

Jessica: "I can eat an apple for snack, and we could make a salad with some chicken for dinner once in a while."

Nurse: "That sounds great, Jessica. Why don't you and your parents look for some fun meals you can make at home and set a target for eating an apple every day for a snack and making two meals at home a week rather than getting takeout? I can give you a calendar to help track your progress."

Mom: "We can do that."

Nurse: "Let's check in again in 2 weeks to see how things are going and make any changes if needed."

This approach is very typical and involves education and planning. It has many supportive and effective techniques we could break down, such as listening to Jessica and her family and the challenges they have faced. The nurse also asked for input from the family, including Jessica, to incorporate into the plan. Let's compare this same situation and incorporate MI into the NGN process and see how that feels.

NGN Approach with Motivational Interviewing

We will go through the steps of the NGN process, but we will use the MI techniques we have talked about for conversation.

Step 1: Recognize cues (assessment): The nurse gathers subjective and objective data about Jessica's situation while using MI techniques to engage Jessica and her mother.

> *Nurse* (engaging): "Hi, Jessica. Hi, Mrs. Smith. I know the past year has been tough for many families, and it sounds like you've had a lot of changes to adjust to. Can you tell me a little about what your days have been like recently?"
>
> *Jessica*: "I've been doing school on Zoom and playing video games. I don't really go outside much."
>
> *Nurse* (reflective listening): "It sounds like you've been spending a lot of time indoors and on screens. That's been common for kids during the pandemic. What do you like most about your current routine?"
>
> *Jessica*: "I like playing games, but I miss playing soccer with my friends."
>
> *Nurse* (recognizing cues toward change talk): "So, you enjoy video games, but you also miss being active and spending time with your friends. That's helpful to know. Mrs. Smith, how has your family's routine changed over the past year?"
>
> *Mother*: "Well, I work evenings, and my husband works during the day, so we've been relying on fast food a lot. It's easier when we're so busy."
>
> *Nurse* (empathy): "That makes sense. It sounds like you've been juggling a lot, and fast food has been a convenient option."

Step 2: Analyze cues and prioritize hypotheses (Analysis): The nurse interprets the data to identify Jessica's health risks and prioritizes hypotheses about the barriers to a healthier lifestyle.

> *Nurse* (evoking change talk): "From what you've shared, it seems like the main challenges are finding time for physical activity and preparing healthier meals. Does that sound right?"
>
> *Mother*: "Yes, it's hard to find time to cook, and Jessica doesn't really want to go outside much anymore."

Nurse (prioritizing hypotheses): "Okay, so it sounds like we need to focus on two things: helping Jessica get back to being active in a way she enjoys and finding easy, healthy meal options that work for your family's schedule."

Step 3: Generate solutions (planning): The nurse collaborates with Jessica and her mother to develop a plan, using MI techniques to evoke Jessica's motivation and involve her in the decision-making process.

Nurse (evoking): "Jessica, you mentioned that you miss playing soccer with your friends. What do you think you could do to start that up again?"

Jessica: "Yeah, I think I'd like to play soccer again. Maybe I could start by just kicking the ball around."

Nurse (planning): "That's a great idea!"

Nurse (collaborating with the family): "Mrs. Smith, for meals, what are your thoughts about trying some quick, healthy options, like precut veggies or rotisserie chicken? We could also talk about ways to make fast-food choices a little healthier when you're short on time, if that is something you want to explore."

Mother: "I'm thinking I could get some more fresh fruit and maybe try crockpot meals, so my husband does not have to prepare anything."

Step 4: Act (implementation): The nurse supports Jessica and her family in implementing the plan, using MI techniques to reinforce their confidence and commitment.

Nurse (supporting empowerment): "Jessica, it sounds like you're excited to start playing soccer again. How confident do you feel about playing outside a few times this week, on a scale from 1 to 10?"

Jessica: "Maybe a 7."

Nurse: "That's a great start! What would make it an 8 or 9?"

Jessica: "If my friend could come over to play with me."

Nurse: "That's a great idea. Let's see if you can invite a friend to join you. And Mrs. Smith, how confident do you feel about trying some of those quick meal ideas?"

Mother: "I think I could do it. Maybe an 8."

Nurse: "That's wonderful. Remember, small changes can make a big difference. I'll check in with you next week to see how things are going."

Step 5: Evaluate outcomes (evaluation): The nurse follows up with Jessica and her family to assess progress and adjust the plan as needed.

Nurse (evaluating outcomes): "Hi, Jessica. Hi, Mrs. Smith. How did things go this week? Jessica, were you able to play outside like we talked about?"

Jessica: "Yeah, I played soccer with my friend twice. It was fun!"

Nurse: "That's fantastic! How did you feel afterward?"

Jessica: "I felt good. I wasn't as tired as I thought I'd be."

Nurse: "That's great to hear. Let's keep building on that. Mrs. Smith, how did the meal changes go?"

Mother: "We tried some crock pot meals twice and Jessica even helped me prepare them."

Nurse: "That's amazing! It sounds like you're both making great progress. Let's set some new goals for next week to keep things moving forward."

Questions to Discuss

Think about the following questions:

- Did you notice a difference in how the two scenarios were different?
- Which one did you like better? Why or why not?
- Which one empowered the patient and her family to make changes?
- Which one do you think they will act on when they go home? Why or why not?

Let's look at some of the reasons the second scenario might have resonated more with you by breaking down each step and looking at the techniques that were used as well as the results they produced.

- *Recognizing cues* (NGN): The nurse needs to gather information about the patient's situation, identify any relevant data, and recognize a pattern or cue that may indicate a problem. By utilizing MI techniques such as open-ended questions, the patient will provide this detailed information. For example, "Jessica, can you tell me about what your days have been like recently? What kinds of things do you enjoy doing?" This question fosters a relationship and shows the patient you are interested in what they think. It allows the patient to explore what they are feeling and share those feelings with the provider. With reflective listening, you could help to clarify information, especially if you got something wrong such as "It sounds like you've been spending a lot of time indoors and playing video games because it's been hard to go outside." In this way, the patient can correct any misconceptions or reflect on what you just said as being accurate.

- *Analyzing cues*: The nurse in this step interprets the cues to identify patterns, relationships, or potential problems. Summarizing is a technique that can help the nurse organize and reflect on all the information gathered: "So, from what you've shared, it seems like the pandemic has made it harder to stay active, and fast food has become a regular part of your meals. Does that sound right?" Again, the patient can correct any misconceptions or agree this is an accurate assessment. Developing discrepancy is another technique that can help patients see a gap between what they want and what they are doing. For example, "You mentioned that you miss playing soccer with your friends and feeling more energetic. How do you think your current routine is affecting your energy levels?" This statement is nonthreatening yet causes a person to pause and reflect on the discrepancy.
- *Prioritizing hypothesis*: At this stage, the nurse determines which problems or issues need to be addressed based on the cues and the analysis, but with MI the solutions will come from the patient not the nurse. For example, in eliciting change talk you try to get the patient to express their own reasons for wanting to make a change and help them to prioritize their most meaningful goals. A question such as "What do you think would be the most important change for you to feel healthier and more energetic?" puts the ball in their court. You are not suggesting a plan or telling them what they need to do, you are asking them what is most important to them. That may seem like a small change, but it is a huge shift in perspective. Exploring ambivalence is another technique recognizes that patients are many times ambivalent to change. For example, "On one hand, you enjoy playing video games, but on the other, you miss being active and spending time with your friends. What feels most important to you right now?" Again, this is a vastly different approach, one that will cause the patient to reflect on what they really think or want to do.
- *Generating solutions*: Now you will brainstorm with your patient to come up with interventions or solutions that will address the prioritized problems. With MI, the goal is to set small achievable measurable goals, which go hand in hand with SMART goals. Asking the patient "What is one small step you feel ready to take this week? Maybe going for a short walk after dinner or trying a new recipe with your mom or dad?" Affirmations can go

a long way when they come up with some solutions. For example, "It's great you're thinking about ways to be more active. You've already taken the first step by coming here and talking about it."

- *Acting*: The nurse implements the chosen interventions and supports the patient in taking steps toward the goals they have set. The focus of MI is on empowering patients to believe in their own abilities to make the changes they want to make. This step is critical in the action phase. For example, "You've decided to play soccer again by kicking the ball around outside with your friends. That's a great plan, and I know you can do it." By helping patients set up that plan you show you are really interested in supporting them. For example, "Let's figure out what days and times work best for you to be outside playing. Would it help to set a reminder or plan it around something you already do, like after dinner?"
- *Evaluating outcomes*: How effective were the interventions? Were the goals met? It is important for this step not to feel like going to the principal's office. You must remember this is the patients' plan and the patients' goals and you are not the one responsible for their success. You are there to help support them achieve their goals or refine them whichever the case may be. Reflecting on progress is one way to help patients recognize their achievements. For example, "How did your walks go this week? What went well, and what was challenging?" Based on the answers, reassess and adjust the plan. For example, "If playing soccer after dinner didn't work out, what might be a better time or activity for you? Let's figure out what feels right for you."

Table 6.1 Comparison of NGN and MI Alignment

NGN STEP	MI Technique	Purpose
Recognize cues	Open-ended questions, reflective listening	Gather detailed information and validate the patient's perspective
Analyze cues	Summarizing, developing discrepancy	Identify patterns and help the patient see the gap between current and desired behaviors
Prioritizing hypothesis	Eliciting change talk, exploring ambivalence	Focus on the most meaningful and achievable goals for the patient

NGN STEP	MI Technique	Purpose
Generating solutions	Collaborative goal setting, affirmations	Empower the patient to take steps toward their goals and implement solutions
Taking action	Supporting self-efficacy, planning	Empower the patient to take steps toward their goals and implement solutions
Evaluating outcomes	Reflecting on progress, reassessing and adjusting	Assess effectiveness and make adjustments to the plan as needed

As you can see, the NGN model and MI techniques complement each other well. Both models emphasize patient-centered care, with MI taking it one step further, allowing the patients to drive the care and find their own motivation with your support. Both techniques involve critical thinking skills and a cyclical approach to problem solving in realizing that change is a process that moves forward and backward all the time. Nurses can enhance their ability to engage patients by utilizing MI techniques and address ambivalence, which is much more common than we think. These techniques will help support sustainable behavior change in a way that feels good to the patient by empowering them to make the changes they want in their life in a more meaningful way. Let's turn to the evidence to see what studies say about the effectiveness of MI in nursing practice.

Evidence-Based Practice

A study done by Östlund et al. (2015) sought to understand the experience primary nurses had with utilizing MI after receiving training on it with a qualitative study involving 20 primary care nurses. Nurses expressed their own initial ambivalence to learning something new, such as "It was easier to behave as usual, doing what one should, giving advice," or "What's hard is simply thinking differently … We're so programmed to deliver … well all the advice. We're trained in the expert model." Other comments included a lack of time to utilize the techniques as well as some patients expecting to receive advice and information rather than an exploration of their feelings.

In the end, the nurses agreed that the training was an opportunity for mutual benefits for both patients and nurses. Benefits included empowering patients to find the ability within themselves to make the necessary changes, increasing the nurse's ability to increase patient motivation, and improving their own empathetic ability. Positive statements included "I try to go deeper using scales, asking where they are on them, to find out how I should continue and try to elicit talk about change" and "Make use of their own experiences instead of pushing things on them all the time. That's how we used to work; you give a lot of advice and don't really listen to the patient, so this is a way to listen and its better." The nurses all felt that training in MI was good but that ongoing training with feedback was essential to master the skills, and nurses had to have an interest in wanting to learn these skills (Östlund et al., 2015).

Dray et al. (2014) studied the effects of training mental health nurses on an eating disorder unit in MI to decrease premature discharge from the unit. They wanted to know if brief training in MI could have a positive effect. Six nurses who worked on the unit were trained in MI, and their treatment adherence and competence were evaluated post-training and at a 2-month follow-up. Pre- and postimplementation rates on premature discharge rates were compared at the conclusion of the study, and the results showed that nurses trained in MI showed significant improvement in MI adherence and competence as well as gave high satisfaction scores for the training. Patients also were well satisfied with the MI intervention, and premature discharge rates significantly decreased postimplementation, showing its effectiveness (Dray et al., 2014).

Chronic disease costs Americans $1.65 trillion annually. Many chronic diseases can be managed effectively with proper medication and/or lifestyle changes. Providers see patients on a regular basis for chronic disease and try to educate and advise them on what they need to do, many times with subpar results. One example of this is a type 2 diabetic in the hospital who within a very short period of time has their blood sugar under control only to find when they go home that it is again out of control. This may seem baffling, but when you think about it, when patients are in the hospital, they eat the diet the way it is prescribed, and they get their blood sugar checked regularly, as well as their medications. The same is true for many other chronic diseases. What happens when they go home? At home patients are in control of the medications they take, many times forgetting to take a dose, and they eat the way they usually do, which may not be anywhere near the way they should.

Minkin et al. (2014) conducted a survey on veterans who were home bound in medication adherence rate utilizing an MI intervention as opposed to no MI intervention. The number of veterans enrolled in home visits varied between 150 to 200 patients, with an average of 178 veterans enrolled during the study period. The design was a retrospective chart review both pre- and postimplementation of the MI intervention. Nurses (RN/LPNs) were trained by a psychologist for 4 hours in MI techniques, and there were weekly share sessions with feedback for 6 months. Medication was analyzed for compliance, Warfarin specifically because it requires close monitoring and is frequently prescribed in this population. The results of the study were as follows: Overall medication adherence at 6 months preimplementation was 22.3%, 1-month postimplementation was 13.1%, and at 6 months postimplementation was 14.0%. Warfarin-specific adherence at 6 months preimplementation was 22.2%, 1-month postimplementation was 22.7%, and at 6 months postimplementation was 12.8%. These results confirm that an MI intervention can significantly improve medication adherence rates, which subsequently will improve chronic disease management. The results also show that MI is a perfect fit for a home nursing situation, when a long-term trusting relationship will ensue. The role of the nurse in this case was to facilitate rather than educate or dictate, creating a more patient-driven collaborative approach (Minkin et al., 2014).

Real-Life Case Studies

Nurses engage with patients in multiple ways and have ample opportunity to introduce MI techniques in their daily interactions with patients. Nurses are also not generally seen as the authoritative figure; the provider is, which makes a better fit for this technique. Let's look at what a real-life scenario might look like utilizing an opportunity to use MI between a nurse and a patient.

- Patient: Mr. Smith, 52 years old, admitted for chest pain with a history of hypertension
- Nurse: Raven, RN trained in MI techniques

Nurse Raven reviews Mr. Smith's chart and sees he is being worked up for acute coronary syndrome, and there is concern he may have some cardiac disease. Nurse Raven understands that smoking has been a contributing factor to the problems that Mr. Smith has with coronary artery disease and begins a conversation with Mr. Smith while performing routine daily care that goes something like this:

Establishing Rapport and Assessing Readiness

> *Nurse Raven*: "Mr. Smith, I see you have been managing your high blood pressure for quite a while now. How have you been feeling about your health lately?"
>
> *Mr. Smith* (shrugs, avoids eye contact): "It's alright, I guess. Just wondering what is going on, trying to keep up with all these pills."
>
> *Nurse Raven* (nods, maintains open body language): "It sounds like it can be a lot to manage. I also noticed you've been smoking for some time. Would it be okay if we talked a bit about that?"
>
> *Mr. Smith* (sighs, looks away): "Yeah, I know it is not good for me. I wish I could quit but it helps with stress, you know."

Nurse Raven (reflective listening): "You're aware of the risks, but smoking feels like it helps you cope with stress." (Notice here how Nurse Raven has picked up on Mr. Smith's ambivalence. He knows smoking is bad for his health on one hand, but he gets benefits such as stress reduction on the other hand.)

Exploring Ambivalence and Eliciting Change Talk

Nurse Raven: "Many people I talk to feel the same way. They know that smoking is bad for them on the one hand but can't imagine life without it. What are some things you like about smoking, and what are some things you don't like?"

Mr. Smith: "Well, it calms me down; it's like a little reward for a job well done when I take a break. I feel like, as crazy as it sounds, I can take a deep breath and just relax. Maybe it's the menthol or just my mind playing tricks on me. I don't know, but I don't like the cough in the morning, and I have noticed I get short of breath easily lately. My wife's been on me to quit for years."

Nurse Raven (affirmation): "It takes a lot of honesty to talk about both sides. You're noticing the impact it's having on your health and your relationship." (In this case Nurse Raven is using open-ended questions and affirmations, key MI techniques, to encourage Mr. Smith to express his own motivations and concerns.)

Responding to Cues and Supporting Autonomy

Nurse Raven: "On one hand, smoking helps with stress, and on the other, you're worried about your health and your wife's concerns. Where do you see yourself in terms of wanting to make a change?" (Notice Nurse Raven is letting the decision to quit be up to Mr. Smith and is not instructing him that he should quit.)

Mr. Smith (leans forward, makes eye contact): "I've thought about quitting, but I'm not sure I can do it. I've tried before and it didn't stick."

Nurse Raven (reflective listening and supporting self-efficacy): "You've tried before, which shows you're capable of making changes, even if it's tough. What do you think made it hard to stick with the last time?" (Nurse Raven noticed the change in body language (leaning forward, making eye contact), a nonverbal cue indicating increased engagement and possible readiness to discuss change.)

Collaborative Planning and Summarizing

Mr. Smith: "I get irritable, and then I just go back to it. Maybe if I had more support or some medication that would help, I could try again, I guess. It seems like I can do it when I am in the hospital."

Nurse Raven: "Quitting smoking is a hard thing to do and having support can make a big difference. If you decide you want to try quitting again, I can help connect you with resources such as support groups or nicotine replacement options. Would you be interested in hearing more about those options, or would you prefer to think about it for now?"

Mr. Smith: "Maybe just some information for now. I'll think about it."

Nurse Raven (summarizing and leaving the door open): "Absolutely, today we talked about smoking and how you feel both ways about it. One the one hand it brings you some stress relief, and on the other you see how it is impacting your life. You have tried to quit before but were not successful in your attempt. You would like to quit but feel you need more support and maybe some medication. I'll leave some information here for you, and if you want to talk more about it, I'm here to help. You're in control of when and how you want to make any changes in your life." (Nurse Raven summarized the conversation, respects Mr. Smith's autonomy, and leaves the door open for future discussion, consistent with MI principles.)

Key MI Techniques Demonstrated

- Open-ended questions: To explore Mr. Smith's feelings and motivations
- Reflective listening: To validate his experience
- Developing discrepancies: Pointing out ambivalence
- Affirmations: To build confidence and rapport
- Summarizing: To reinforce key points and support autonomy
- Responding to verbal and nonverbal cues (e.g., avoidance, engagement): To tailor the conversation and pace

Notice how this technique did not involve educating Mr. Smith on the dangers of smoking and did not try to scare him with facts about how smoking could cause him to die prematurely. Think about why this conversation went better than the educational or expert approach and what you liked more about it.

KEY POINTS

- Nursing is an art form that involves connecting with patients during some of their most intense and vulnerable times and involves blending the art of science with the art of empathy and compassion.
- Nurses are well suited to integrate MI skills into ordinary conversations when they interact with patients.
- MI skills blend well with the nursing process.
- MI in regard to lifestyle changes is an evidence-based skill.

QUESTIONS FOR REFLECTION

- How can I use motivational interviewing (MI) as a tool within my nursing scope of practice to help facilitate patient behavior change?
- In what ways do the frequent and extended interactions I have with patients create opportunities for meaningful conversations about their health behaviors?
- How might integrating MI techniques into each step of the nursing process enhance patient engagement and improve health outcomes?
- What strategies can I use to foster a more collaborative and satisfying care experience for my patients through the use of MI?
- How does utilizing MI contribute to an evidence-based approach to supporting lifestyle changes in the nursing process?

SUGGESTED ACTIVITIES

1. Role-playing scenarios: Organize role-playing sessions during which nursing students can practice MI skills in various situations.
2. Reflective journaling: Have students' journal their attempts at utilizing MI skills in patient encounters and talk about these experiences in groups.

References

Dray, J., Gilchrist, P., Singh, D., Cheesman, G., & Wade, T. (2014). Training mental health nurses to provide motivational interviewing on an inpatient eating disorder unit. *Journal of Psychiatric and Mental Health Nursing, 21*(7), 652–657. https://doi.org/10.1111/jpm.12163

Minkin, A., Snider-Meyer, J., Olson, D., Gresser, S., Smith, H., & Kier, F. J. (2014). Effectiveness of a motivational interviewing intervention on medication compliance. *Home Healthcare Nurse*, *32*(8), 490–496. https://doi.org/10.1097/nhh.0000000000000128

Östlund, A.-S., Wadensten, B., Kristofferzon, M.-L., & Häggström, E. (2015). Motivational interviewing: Experiences of primary care nurses trained in the method. *Nurse Education in Practice*, *15*(2), 111–118. https://doi.org/10.1016/j.nepr.2014.11.005

Peplau, H. E. (1988). The art and science of nursing: Similarities, differences, and relations. *Nursing Science Quarterly*, *1*(1), 8–15. https://doi.org/10.1177/089431848800100105

Chapter 7

Advanced Practice Application

However beautiful the strategy is, you should occasionally look at the results.

—Winston Churchill

We have known for a long time that MI works in counseling sessions and was initially developed as a collaborative, goal-orientated technique aimed at strengthening an individual's motivation for change specifically as it relates to tobacco and alcohol use. In this chapter, we will explore how MI is being used in primary care to improve health with chronic health conditions such as obesity, hypertension, coronary artery disease, diabetes, and vaccine hesitancy, as well as the experience providers describe with learning MI techniques and implementing MI into their practice.

OBJECTIVES

- Students will be able to analyze and summarize key findings in studies that show how MI can improve outcomes in primary care as an evidence-based modality.
- Students will be able to evaluate the impact MI had on behaviors such as vaccine hesitancy, weight management, or managing chronic health conditions.
- Students will be able to identify common barriers patients have with behavior change and discuss how MI utilizes an approach that is more acceptable.

KEY TERMS AND DEFINITIONS

- **Vaccine resistance**: A person who has made up their mind and decided against vaccination.
- **Vaccine hesitancy**: A person who is hesitant but willing to discuss getting vaccinated.
- **Patient empowerment**: The process whereby patients gain knowledge, skills, and confidence to manage their own health and make informed decisions.
- **Chronic disease management**: A comprehensive approach to managing chronic diseases, many of which include lifestyle changes.

We have discussed at length what MI is and some of the techniques that are involved in learning it, and we know it works for counseling, but the question is "Does it *really work* in primary care, and if so, how well?" Primary care providers deal with the entire medical management of the patient. They cover acute and **chronic disease management** as well as health promotion. From the earliest days of our life, we begin with well visits from childhood through adulthood. Preventive visits become less frequent but are still encouraged as we age. As adults we may find ourselves visiting our primary care providers more often as we age.

Primary care providers develop a long-term relationship with patients and their families and under ideal circumstances a trusting one. This setting is the perfect medium for MI skills. Approaching patients in a nonjudgmental authentic way is what the spirit of MI is all about. Primary care providers encounter patients who are ambivalent to change all the time. In the following sections we will examine some common issues in primary care and look at the research that supports an MI approach.

MI and Evidence-Based Practice

Vaccinations

A common area in primary care dealing directly with health promotion is vaccinations. Correcting misconceptions is a big part of being a primary care provider. There is a difference between **vaccine resistance** and **vaccine hesitancy**, and we should take a minute to define the difference. A *vaccine-resistant* person has done their own research, and they have concluded that they do not want vaccines for various reasons. Usually, they are not open to talking about them and giving them more "education" does not work; in fact, it may be viewed by some to be offensive. *Vaccine-hesitant* persons are more open to discussing things and depending on the approach you take you might be more successful. An important first step to remember is that before you can have any conversation with a patient, they must first feel like they have been heard and that their opinion matters (Breckenridge et al., 2021).

Before 1960, there was not a nationwide vaccination program. In 1962, the Vaccination Assistance Act (VAA) began. This gave the CDC the ability to initiate mass national vaccination campaigns, and it laid the foundation for federal financial support of them. In the 1960s, the recommended vaccinations for children up to 6 years of age included the diphtheria, tetanus, and pertussis (DTP) vaccine with subsequent boosters; the polio vaccine; and the smallpox vaccine. In total about six vaccinations were given before the child entered school (The Truth About Vaccines, 2025). Compare that to today when over 36 vaccines are recommend before the age of 6, and one can see why parents may be hesitant about vaccinating their children. Inaccurate information about the safety of vaccinations did not help matters and can be a significant barrier. In 1998, a report came out in a scientific journal that linked autism to the measles, mumps, and rubella (MMR) vaccine. Although the journal later retracted the article, and several subsequent scientific studies proved the data to be inaccurate, the damage had been done (DeStefano & Shimabukuro, 2019). Many parents became hesitant or outright resistant to their children receiving the MMR vaccine after that, and for some that belief has persisted for over 20 years.

In the knowledge age, patients and their care givers can gain access to both reliable and unreliable information through the internet. Providers find themselves trying to educate and correct misconceptions during well visits when vaccinations are recommended, taking the approach that they will correct misconceptions with education, provide strong recommendations to vaccinate, and convince parents to vaccinate their children. Many providers feel caught in the middle between recommending what science claims to be best for children and honoring parental wishes. Common themes parents cited as reasons for not wanting to vaccinate their children include safety concerns to include fear of autism, pain and discomfort, lack of necessity, and giving multiple vaccinations all at one time. Studies have shown that although parents trust providers the most for information, education alone does not seem to improve their uptake (Garcia & O'Leary, 2020). A study by Nyhan et al. (2014) looked at the effect of four different types of education regarding vaccinations and the subsequent results. One group of parents received information dispelling the belief with scientific evidence that the MMR vaccine causes autism, another group was educated on the dangers of an infection with MMR, and yet another group was shown images of MMR, with the last group being given a narrative on an infant who almost died from a measles infection. The results showed that *none* of these educational measures were effective at changing the intent of parents to immunize their children.

Looking for a better way Gagneur et al. (2018) developed an approach called PromoVac, which entailed teaching research nurses' theory and techniques on MI delivered to parents in a postpartum maternity ward. The study involved 3,300 parents and was a randomized control trial (RCT). The intervention was brief, lasting only 15 to 20 minutes, with simple direct conversations that allowed for questions and feedback rather than the educational approach previously tried. The model they used was Prochaska's stages of change, which acknowledges that people can pass through several stages before they make a change in behavior. The MI intervention was adapted to the parents' readiness for vaccination. The research nurses touched on five different points throughout the discussion involving how diseases are prevented by vaccines, how effective vaccines are, the importance of the schedule, concerns that vaccines might pose, and the organization of the vaccine services. Results from this study showed that 15% more parents intended to get their children vaccinated at 2 months than prior to the intervention, and there was a 9% overall increase in completion of vaccination from 0–2 years in this group (Gagneur et al., 2018). These results were repeated in a provincial RCT, resulting in a 12% intention to vaccinate with a 40% reduction in vaccine hesitancy utilizing the same technique and showing that approaching parents in the maternity ward prior to the 2-month visit was beneficial. Using an MI approach and taking time to listen to parents, acknowledge their concerns, and give information *as solicited* allowed parents to make a more informed decision regarding their children and was more successful than just an educational approach.

COVID brought with it a new set of issues when it came to public health, trust, and vaccinations. Government mandates and interference were seen by many as a threat to their autonomy and created a whole new set of people with vaccine hesitancy for different reasons. Data suggests that for minority populations and those of low socioeconomic status COVID-19 hit the hardest. It has also been identified that in these groups there was the highest rate of COVID-19 hesitancy (Breckenridge et al., 2021). COVID-19 was a novel disease and progressed rapidly with devastating results. The push for a vaccine was urgent and expediated. The political climate was ripe for concern, and many people, including health care workers, were leery of the vaccine and talked amongst themselves and spread information both good and bad on the internet. Answers to why natural immunity did not negate the need for a vaccine, how long the vaccine would last, or the side effects from the vaccine were legitimate, and the answers we got to those questions were confusing and conflicted. By June of 2021 only 42% of adults in the United States had been vaccinated for COVID-19 (Brecknaridge et al., 2021). Brecknaridge et al. (2021) suggest that utilizing an MI approach with COVID-19 vaccines might be more effective with uptake. They point out that the cornerstone of MI is **patient empowerment**, and that was what was severely lacking in this case. They suggest the approach to vaccine-hesitant patients with COVID-19 includes utilizing the OARS technique. Open-ended questions allow health care workers to explore with patients their fears and concerns rather than just provide education. By letting patients tell their story, the conversation begins in a nonjudgmental way that allows the patient to feel heard. By affirming that patients have legitimate concerns and that we do not have all the answers would build trust. Reflecting with empathy and sensitivity would allow patients to reflect on the advantages and disadvantages of taking the COVID-19 vaccine. Summarizing what had been said during the conversation would serve to strengthen the relationship, validating that the decision to vaccinate or not was up to the patient.

Asking for permission to share more information was also an important step. No one likes unsolicited advice, ever. By utilizing these techniques, providers could begin to build a bridge of understanding that could allow the patient to explore emotionally charged topics without feeling threatened or dismissed. Breckenridge et al. (2021) point out that MI has a growing body of evidence showing that it works to decrease vaccine hesitancy for many other vaccines and may be the better approach with COVID-19, pointing out that training in MI is imperative for health care providers as early in their careers as possible.

Another framework worthy of mention is "What Matters to You?" (WMTY). This person-centered communication style aligns with the spirit of MI. Barry and Edgman-Levitan (2012) first discussed this technique in a *New England Journal of Medicine* (NEJM) article on shared decision-making. The movement has now become a global one and has spread across 50 countries. With this method the idea is to find out the *why*. The idea is to ask the patient what matters to them the most, then listen to what they tell you, and then do what matters most for them by partnering with the patient and incorporating what you have learned about them into the plan of care. This aligns with the simple four-step MI-based framework developed by Gagneur et al. (2024) as a method to approach vaccine-hesitant conversations:

1. Engage/establish trust (safe space).
2. Understand views (find out what matters to them).
3. Offer information (target what matters—ask permission to give information, give them information, then ask if they have questions).
4. Clarify and accept their decision (autonomy; Gagneur et al., 2024).

Obesity

Obesity was recognized as a disease by the American Medical Association (AMA) in 2013 to promote more research and treatment options to treat it (Fryhofer, 2013). Obesity has been associated with up to 60 comorbidities. Yet, policy and treatment options remain limited, with suboptimal insurance coverage for effective treatment. The American Heart Association found that approximately one third of U.S. adults have obesity as do 17% of children aged 2 through 19 (Rosen, 2014). Obesity involves *lifestyle changes,* including diet and exercise, which makes MI an excellent option for providers to consider utilizing with patients suffering from it. Let's look at several populations, starting with the pediatric population, and see how MI was utilized. Woolford et al. (2022) studied the cost-effectiveness of a 2-year MI intervention in a pediatric setting verses usual primary care. The age of the children was between 2 and 8 years of age with a BMI percentile between 85% and 97%; 312 children were included in the analysis, and after 2 years 72% of the enrolled parent/child dyads were retained. According to Woolford et al. (2022), few primary care interventions targeting pediatric obesity have been successful, except for a brief MI intervention to reduce child BMI study, which showed statistically significant decreases in BMI in children between 2 and 8 over a 2-year period. This study consisted of a three-arm RCT, with one group consisting of primary care providers and registered dieticians who received MI training; children in this group saw the primary care provider (PCP) four times in a 2-year period and had six sessions with a registered dietician (RD) over the same time period. The other group included only the PCP visits, and the final group had usual care. Only the PCP/RD group showed statistically significant decreases in BMI. However, given these sessions were brief and only totaled 10 over 24 months, some of which were on the phone, they still made a statistically significant impact. Woolford et al. (2022) did a cost analysis of this study and found it to be cost-effective, concluding that more training for providers and registered dietitians in this technique should be done to combat childhood obesity.

Lutaud et al. (2023) did a systematic literature review of MI for the management of childhood and adolescent obesity. They reviewed 444 articles and identified 26 RCT. They found significant results for all criteria in both children and adolescents with subsequent improvement in depression and quality of life scores. It appears from these studies that for children parental presence is important. Their conclusion states that MI is a promising framework for the obesity problem in this population. Another study by Resnicow et al. (2024) tried to replicate these results by randomizing 18 pediatric primary care practices to implement a brief MI intervention to reduce BMI protocol and found no statistical significance; however, it was also conducted on an older age group of children between 3 and 11years of age. It was also conducted during the height of COVID, which could have impacted the results significantly.

A qualitative study was done by Lindhardt et al. (2015) that included 11 providers trained in MI who had been practicing the technique for 18 months. The participants were obese pregnant women. The results were positive, with all providers stating the MI communication technique was useful, but providers had to be dedicated to it. Time constraints were an issue. However, most health care professionals felt it helped them be more professional. They were more at ease introducing the topic of obesity by asking permission to talk about it and felt it was an overall good experience.

Diabetes

Diabetes involves multiple lifestyle changes and monitoring. In a parallel group blind RCT conducted by İşleyen et al. (2025), 70 participants were recruited (36 in the intervention group and 34 in the control group). Inclusion criteria included being over the age of 18, being on insulin or insulin plus oral therapy, having a diagnosis of diabetes type 2 (DMT2) for at least 1 year, having BMI of

25 or more, having a HbA1c at 7% or above, and having access to a phone. The intervention included four sessions with a nurse trained in MI through telenursing. The total time for the phone call was between 45 and 60 minutes. Results showed improvement in self-care management and efficacy, decreases in fasting blood glucose and triglycerides, and a significant decrease in hemoglobin A1c, supporting further training in public health nursing on MI techniques.

Dineen et al. (2022) did a qualitative review to understand the successes and challenges from a MI-informed diabetes prevention program that was situated in a community. Participants included 14 clients and 10 trainers in a 9-month program. Results found benefit in MI techniques for both clients and trainers, which resulted in the clients making diet and exercise modifications. Challenges were that trainers found learning MI to be challenging and required ongoing effort. With practice the use of the skills became more intuitive. Recommendations included ongoing skills training in MI.

Fall Prevention

Falling can be a huge risk for adult patients, with subsequent injury and hospitalizations leading to increased mortality the older we get. However, older adults do not consistently practice fall prevention strategies to the dismay of their providers. Adherence to fall prevention strategies is estimated to be 34 to 52%. Part of the reason for this nonadherence is the belief that they are not at risk of falling despite the aging process. MI has been used to improve adherence to fall prevention strategies. A pilot study was conducted by Kiyoshi-Teo et al. (2024) to determine if an MI strategy could improve adherence to fall prevention strategies. The pilot study was a RCT and consisted of 200 participants with a mean age of 80 years; 67% were female. MI was conducted virtually via a telephone call due to the COVID-19 pandemic. The results of the study were favorable but may have been impacted by the pandemic. Once lockdown was lifted there was less participation from the intervention group, resulting in no significant change between the groups. Recommendations included that further studies should be conducted with more favorable conditions to determine if MI can effectively engage older adults in fall prevention strategies, decreasing their fall risk (Kiyoshi-Teo et al., 2024).

Physical Activity

Increasing physical activity can have a profound influence on your health. Many chronic diseases can be improved by just moving more, with seven out of 10 chronic diseases showing improvement with increased activity (U.S. Department of Health and Human Services, 2024). PCPs advocate for their patients to sit less and move more. Evidence shows that MI is a positive strategy to help people define their goals better and adopt a physical activity plan that improves their health and meets their goals. According to a study by Hardcastle et al. (2012) involving 207 patients who were offered MI sessions to support activity behavior change within a deprived community, we saw positive results. In this study, qualified providers referred patients to a "lifestyle change facilitation service" whereby they received MI sessions. Patients who were enrolled were either sedentary or insufficiently to moderately active, and there were no physical limitations. MI skills were utilized and incorporated into the transtheoretical stages of change model. Participants were not educated on why they should move more or told reasons they needed to change. The focus was on their ambivalence, listening for change talk and readiness, exploring the pluses and minuses of change, agenda setting, and once participants showed interest in changing building on that. Strategies included questioning such as "On a scale of 1–10 (with 10 being the highest), how important is it for you to increase your physical activity level?" Each session was individualized, and at 6 months significant increases could be seen in physical activity, including vigorous activity, stage of change, and support systems from baseline, which supports previous research in this regard (Hardcastle et al., 2012).

Hyperlipidemia

Hyperlipidemia is a precursor to coronary artery disease. Cardiac disease is the leading cause of death in America. Eating a heart-healthy diet can be challenging in the American culture. In a study by Bóveda-Fontán et al. (2015) involving 25 community health centers, including 38 general practitioners and 227 patients, a RCT was evaluated. The study compared standard care versus an MI approach to decrease lipid levels. Patients were either assigned to the experimental group, which consisted of 107 patients, or the control group, which consisted of 120 patients. Both groups showed a statistically significant reduction in all lipid parameters, cardiovascular risk, weight reduction, and adherence to a Mediterranean diet, with the experimental group who received the MI intervention achieving superior results in combined lipid control with increased physical activity.

Cancer Screening

Finding cancer at an early treatable stage is the goal of most health care professionals. At every visit most providers go over all the different screening recommendations a patient has. MI has been shown to increase the likelihood of a patient's willingness to undergo screening. A study by Chan and So (2021) showed the effectiveness of a brief face-to-face interview or telephone interview utilizing an MI technique. They conducted a systematic literature review, using four databases including a manual search. They only included RCTs that were looking at the effects of MI among average risk patients regarding cancer screening. The results of six RCTs showed that there was an increased uptake for breast and cervical cancer screening but that more studies needed to be conducted regarding other types of cancer screenings.

Another study by Pourebrahim-Alamdari et al. (2022) showed the same results for cervical cancer screening after a brief face-to-face or telephone MI approach for cervical cancer screening on a small group of 150 woman, in Tabriz, Iran, with the recommendations that MI techniques be utilized for cancer screening discussions.

Colorectal cancer screening can be met with resistance from patients. Many patients fear the prep or do not want to undergo an invasive procedure. They have questions and often will delay screening because of that. Wahab et al. (2008) studied the effects of an MI technique delivered by a trained interventionist in MI via a telephone counseling session. They found that 20.5% of MI participants reported having a CRC screening test with another 19.75% scheduling a screening test after the interview. Approximately 43% of participants reported after the intervention that the telephone call helped them address the barriers that had previously prevented them from completing a screening test.

Implications for practice discuss the need for ongoing supervision and training in the techniques, stating they are "crucial" to support MI fidelity. A particular focus of this study was the training of interventionalists. The interventionalists had a 2-day training session followed by one-on-one testing with an MI specialist to assess readiness for the study. One participant had to receive extra training to be qualified. A telephone interviewing prompt was developed to go through the stages of the MI process, with most interventionalists referring to it at first, but found the prop to be distracting later in the study. One recommendation included ongoing training with weekly sessions to help them hone their skills as they found it was easy to fall back into previously learned patterns.

Lifestyle Changes

At every visit during the intake most providers ask about smoking, drinking, and drug use. We are also encouraged to give brief counseling for these habits as they are at the root cause of many chronic diseases and a leading cause of death in the United States. Usually, the conversation begins with asking patients if they have thought about quitting the habit, if they understand the benefits of quitting, and if they are ready to make that change. In our example, we might say things such as if you quit smoking, you will breathe better, you will have more money to spend, and/or you may live longer. Patients have often come to us for years and have heard the same message repeatedly and really don't want to discuss it. Over time if we fail to convince them to make these changes we may resort to more direct tactics, such as if you don't quit smoking, you could get cancer and die, even going so far as to show them pictures of smoke-affected lungs. Damara Gutnick, an assistant professor of medicine and psychiatry at NYU Langone Medical Center, created a video to discuss an experience with one of her patients over a 15-year time frame and how her approach changed after learning about and receiving training in MI with the subsequent result worth noting. It is worth watching (youtube.com/watch?v=0z65EppMfHk).

In a study by Ridner et al. (2014), utilizing an MI approach with patients regarding smoking cessation resulted in participants becoming less dependent on nicotine with more self-confidence and an increase in patient satisfaction. This result was further increased if the nurse, also trained in MI, did a follow-up call to check in to see how they were doing.

The MI approach can work for any type of addition. Think of something you as a provider love to do and how hard that would be for you to give up. If that habit was attached to negative social connotations such as smoking, drinking, promiscuous behavior, or drug addictions, how much more hesitant would it be for you to bring up the subject to your provider. Brief alcohol counseling techniques utilizing MI are being taught in many practices across the country and are being met with success. One such program is the Michigan Sustained Patient Centered Alcohol Related Care (MI-SPARC; michigansparc.org/src/assets/pdf/MISPARC_Implementation_Guide.pdf).

Provider Perceptions

We know that MI is an effective technique, and we know that providers can benefit from training in it, but how do providers feel about it? Aujoulat et al. (2025) did a qualitative study involving 11 general practitioners (GPs) conducting semi-structured interviews to see how they felt about MI in practice, including the benefits and barriers. Most felt MI could be beneficial in their practice but saw time constraints and training to be the biggest barriers. However, once MI is learned and becomes part of the practitioner's practice it becomes a time saver, with one GP commenting, "If it's a good tool, the situations that may seem time-consuming to us at the start can be much more effective in subsequent consultations so we can make a big gain out of it I think," and another stating "Yes, it can be time consuming, but in a way, 'losing' a little time now could allow me to save time later during other consultations," and with yet another participant recognizing how providers themselves may be resistant to change by stating, "We ask patients to change all the time but, it is us who find it difficult to change" (Aujoulat et al., 2025, p. 6).

Langlois and Goudreau (2022a) conducted research with the aim of studying the clinician's transformation while learning MI skills to see what the barriers were to suboptimal implementation in practice. Sixteen PCPs were recruited, with 12 being involved in the final analysis. These clinicians received formal MI training in four separate sessions totaling 76 hours of training and follow-up focus groups for a total of 8 more hours. Findings included that participants rarely did active listening prior to MI training with their patients. One participant stated, "Before, for the multimorbid patient, I used to tell myself, 'I have my plan, and we will cover hypertension first.' Now I skip that part. Even if there is a lot to cover, my first question is, what brings you in today? What is most important to you? What do you want to work on today and what would you like to change?" (Langlois & Gourdreau, 2022a, p. 255). Gradually, as training continued, participants began to realize that patient visits prior to MI training consisted of providing information or education that was not solicited, and it had the opposite effect than what they had intended. Once they realized this a paradigm shift began to occur in the provider going from being a "health expert to a health guide" (Langlois & Goudreau, 2022a, p. 51).

Implementation of MI in Primary Care

Boom et al. (2022) sought to answer the question of what factors facilitated or impeded the successful implementation of MI into primary care once training was complete. They recruited 152 participants, 93 general practitioners, and 59 practice nurses who were all trained in MI and conducted surveys as well as semi-structured interviews to understand the lived experience of those undergoing training. They found 13 factors to be relevant that could be grouped into three themes: not enough time to implement, lack of self-confidence in techniques, and patient factors such as cultural background. For lack of time one participant stated, "If I know I'm running late and three more patients are waiting I usually don't apply it," meaning MI (Boom et al., 2022, p. 3). Others mentioned that to "have someone at work to motivate each other to continue to engage with MI and to keep reflecting on it" was helpful (Boom et al., 2022, p. 5).

Under lack of confidence, it appears that the more providers experimented with MI the more they could see the benefits. For example, one participant stated, "Personally, I thought it was beneficial that it was presented as something that was part of the job. That's why I chose to quickly master it (MI), and then I noticed the results, which were especially eye opening," (Boom et al., 2022, p. 5). Others noticed patients "feel heard and taken seriously" and "it makes them [patients] more aware of their own responsibility regarding their health" (Boom et al., 2022, p. 5). Overall, participants found MI to be useful, with the greatest challenge being implementing or sustaining the change in practice. Recommendations include paying close attention to the factors that affect implementation and having ongoing support and training from the organization until MI becomes second nature.

Ambivalence

Langlois and Goudreau (2022b) studied the implementation process, further noting that training in MI alone does not lead to successful implementation. Providers go through ambivalence just as their patients do. Providers weigh the value of learning a new skill: Is it worth the time? Does it really make a difference? Do I really have the time to implement it effectively? Comments such as "The two-day training (on MI) was a professional revelation! After that, when you go back to the field, in real life, it takes so much time! 'How am I going to do all of this?" You are searching for your words. You weigh everything you say. You feel like you must put on white gloves every time you speak. You are afraid of making a mistake. Implementing MI is quite a puzzle," reflect the incompetence that newly trained providers feel (Langlois & Goudreau, 2022b, p. 264).

Introspection

Introspection comes next when providers begin to reflect on what they have learned and what they are observing in the interactions. Another participant stated, "I realized that what I thought I was doing well, but fundamentally it wasn't the case. I realized that there were much better ways to intervene with patients and work with them to get results to make changes" (Langlois & Goudreau, 2022b, p. 264). Once providers began to talk about their experiences in an authentic way in the share sessions they were able to give and receive feedback, so the trepidation lessoned with time.

Experimentation

When entering the experimentation phase providers began to feel more confident and experimented with their newfound skills. The terror they once felt using it was lessoning, and breakthroughs occurred: "I remember once using a little sentence that made an impact on a patient? It was like … he almost started to cry after I told him something that hit a nerve. I wasn't used to intervening that way, it's a new way of doing things for me. I realized 'Wow, this is working!'" (Langlois & Goudreau, 2022b, p. 265). Another participant saw that time was not the barrier they initially thought it was: "Finally, I see that we are more and more capable, and I realize that it does not take longer. It is even more effective and facilitating for us!" (Langlois & Goudreau, 2022b, p. 265).

Implementation

Sustainable implementation occurred at the end of their study. All the participants were fully engaged and immersed in utilizing MI as a sustainable approach to behavior change. One participant stated, "It's like we are the patients here. We must prepare ourselves before our meetings, we set our goals, we must practice and change our habits! And you [the teacher] … guide us through it all. Changing our lifestyle, changing our professional practice. It's pretty much the same and it takes time" (Langlois & Goudreau, 2022b, p. 265).

Nursing Education Training

Should training in MI be a part of the prelicensure nursing training? We know it is included in the essentials as a counseling technique for advanced practice. We also know the more we use MI the more comfortable we become with it. A national survey involving 112 prelicensure programs across the United States shows that MI training is included in many prelicensure nursing programs, with 41 replying in the affirmative, citing accreditation requirements as the main motivator and 71 reporting not including this training in their curriculum due to lack of knowledge about it (Badowski et al., 2021).

Lifestyle changes remain the cornerstone of health promotion. MI requires a shift in the way we think about our relationship with our patients. If we think about it, MI can become a freeing force for providers, lessoning the burden and responsibility they feel for patient outcomes and helping empower our patients to take control of their own health and their own lives on their own terms. In the next several chapters we will look at what MI training could look like with several practice exercises to help you become more familiar with it.

KEY POINTS

- MI is an evidence-based counseling approach that is effective in primary care.
- MI has been shown to be effective for vaccine hesitancy.
- MI has been shown to be effective for managing chronic conditions such as obesity, DM, HLD, and coronary artery disease.
- MI has helped older adults with fall prevention.
- MI has been shown to help increase physical activity.
- Provider training needs to be supported by the organization and go beyond initial training.
- Providers go through the same stages of ambivalence, introspection, experimentation, and implementation as their patients do when incorporating MI into practice.
- The “What Matters to You?” framework aligns with the spirit of MI.
- Many nursing schools and NP programs across the United States are incorporating training in MI as part of their curriculum.

QUESTIONS FOR REFLECTION

- How might motivational interviewing (MI) techniques change the way you approach conversations with patients who are hesitant or resistant to health recommendations, such as vaccinations or lifestyle changes?
- Reflect on a time when you or someone you know was ambivalent about making a health-related change. How could the principles of MI—such as open-ended questions, affirmations, reflective listening, and summarizing—have influenced the outcome?
- What barriers do you anticipate facing when trying to implement MI in your future nursing practice, and how might you overcome them?
- How does the “What Matters to You?” framework align with your personal philosophy of patient-centered care, and how could you incorporate it into your clinical interactions?

SUGGESTED ACTIVITIES

1. Say this not that:
    a. Give student a list of sayings that are common in the "expert approach."
    b. Ask students to utilize AI to come up with alternative ways of saying the same thing with the MI approach.
2. Ask students to think of something in their life they really want to change. Utilizing AI, ask the agent to create a scenario with this lifestyle change with the MI and expert approaches. Compare and contrast the two approaches and see which one the student preferred. Which one do they feel might be more successful for them to make meaningful changes?
3. Have students reflect on a time when they had a health care encounter with a nurse or provider that went extremely well or one that went bad. What was the difference?
4. Role-play with two students, one playing the nurse/NP and one the patient. Demonstrate different scenarios using the expert approach and the MI approach and ask the class to give feedback on how the different scenarios played out and how they felt about it.
5. Present real-life scenarios when providers or nurses share experiences when MI was successfully implemented and discuss results.

References

Aujoulat, P., Manac'h, A., Le Reste, C., Le Goff, D., Le Reste, J., & Barais, M. (2025). Investigating assumptions in motivational interviewing among general practitioners: A qualitative study. *BMC Primary Care*, *26*(1). https://doi.org/10.1186/s12875-025-02706-3

Badowski, D., Rossler, K. L., Reiland, N., & Gill Gembala, L. (2021). Integration of motivational interviewing within prelicensure nursing programs. *Nurse Educator*, *47*(3), 168–173. https://doi.org/10.1097/nne.0000000000001127

Barry, M. J., & Edgman-Levitan, S. (2012). Shared decision making—the pinnacle of patient-centered care. *New England Journal of Medicine*, *366*(9), 780–781. https://doi.org/10.1056/nejmp1109283

Boom, S. M., Oberink, R., Zonneveld, A. E., van Dijk, N., & Visser, M. M. (2022). Implementation of motivational interviewing in the general practice setting: A qualitative study. *BMC Primary Care*, *23*(1). https://doi.org/10.1186/s12875-022-01623-z

Bóveda-Fontán, J., Barragán-Brun, N., Campiñez-Navarro, M., Pérula-de Torres, L., Bosch-Fontcuberta, J. M., Martín-Álvarez, R., Arbonies-Ortiz, J., Novo-Rodríguez, J., Criado-Larumbe, M., Fernández-García, J., & Martín-Rioboó, E. (2015). Effectiveness of motivational interviewing in patients with dyslipidemia: A randomized cluster trial. *BMC Family Practice*, *16*(1). https://doi.org/10.1186/s12875-015-0370-2

Breckenridge, L., Burns, D., & Nye, C. (2021). The use of motivational interviewing to overcome COVID-19 vaccine hesitancy in primary care settings. *Public Health Nursing*, *39*(3), 618–623. https://doi.org/10.1111/phn.13003

Chan, D. N., & So, W. K. (2021). Effectiveness of motivational interviewing in enhancing cancer screening uptake amongst average-risk individuals: A systematic review. *International Journal of Nursing Studies*, *113*, 103786. https://doi.org/10.1016/j.ijnurstu.2020.103786

DeStefano, F., & Shimabukuro, T. T. (2019). The MMR vaccine and autism. *Annual Review of Virology*, *6*(1), 585–600. https://doi.org/10.1146/annurev-virology-092818-015515

Dineen, T. E., Bean, C., & Jung, M. E. (2022). Successes and challenges from a motivational interviewing-informed diabetes prevention program situated in the community. *Health Promotion Practice*, *25*(2), 274–284. https://doi.org/10.1177/15248399221115066

Fryhofer, S. A. (2013, June). *Report of the Council on Science and Public Health: Is obesity a disease? (CSAPH Report 3-A-13).* American Medical Association. https://www.ama-assn.org/sites/ama-assn.org/files/corp/media-browser/public/about-ama/councils/Council%20Reports/council-on-science-public-health/a13csaph3.pdf

Gagneur, A., Lemaitre, T., Gosselin, V., Farrands, A., Carrier, N., Petit, G., Valiquette, L., & Wals, P. (2018). Promoting vaccination at birth using motivational interviewing techniques improves vaccine intention: The PromoVac strategy. *Journal of Infectious Diseases & Therapy*, *6*(05). https://doi.org/10.4172/2332-0877.1000379

Gagneur, A., Gutnick, D., Berthiaume, P., Diana, A., Rollnick, S., & Saha, P. (2024). From vaccine hesitancy to vaccine motivation: A motivational interviewing-based approach to vaccine counselling. *Human Vaccines & Immunotherapeutics*, *20*(1), 2391625. https://doi.org/10.1080/21645515.2024.2391625

Garcia, T. B., & O'Leary, S. T. (2020). Dismissal policies for vaccine refusal among US physicians: A literature review. *Human Vaccines & Immunotherapeutics*, *16*(5), 1189–1193. https://doi.org/10.1080/21645515.2020.1724742

Hardcastle, S., Blake, N., & Hagger, M. S. (2012). The effectiveness of a motivational interviewing primary-care based intervention on physical activity and predictors of change in a disadvantaged community. *Journal of Behavioral Medicine*, *35*(3), 318–333. https://doi.org/10.1007/s10865-012-9417-1

İşleyen, E., Özdemir, İ., & Yoldemır, Ş. (2025). The effect of tele-nursing based motivational interviewing on self-efficacy, self-management and metabolic control parameters in individuals with type 2 diabetes: Randomized controlled study. *Irish Journal of Medical Science*, *194*(2), 563–573. https://doi.org/10.1007/s11845-025-03916-5

Kiyoshi-Teo, H., Eckstrom, E., Cohen, D. J., De Lima, B., Northrup-Snyder, K., Dieckman, N. F., & Winters-Stone, K. (2024). Motivational interviewing for fall prevention (MI-FP) pilot study: Randomized controlled trial. *Journal of the American Geriatrics Society*, *73*(4), 1210–1218. https://doi.org/10.1111/jgs.19304

Langlois, S., & Goudreau, J. (2022a). "From health experts to health guides": Motivational interviewing learning processes and influencing factors. *Health Education & Behavior*, *51*(2), 251–259. https://doi.org/10.1177/10901981221084271

Langlois, S., & Goudreau, J. (2022b). Motivational interviewing implementation in primary care: A "terrifying challenge" becoming a "professional revelation." *Health Education & Behavior*, *51*(2), 260–269. https://doi.org/10.1177/10901981221139808

Lindhardt, C., Rubak, S., Mogensen, O., Hansen, H., Goldstein, H., Lamont, R. F., & Joergensen, J. (2015). Healthcare professionals experience with motivational interviewing in their encounter with obese pregnant women. *Midwifery, 31*(7), 678–684. https://doi.org/10.1016/j.midw.2015.03.010

Lutaud, R., Mitilian, E., Forte, J., Gentile, G., Reynaud, R., Truffet, C., & Bellanger, T. (2023). Motivational interviewing for the management of child and adolescent obesity: A systematic literature review. *BJGP Open*, *7*(4). https://doi.org/10.3399/bjgpo.2022.0145

Nyhan, B., Reifler, J., Richey, S., & Freed, G. L. (2014). Effective messages in vaccine promotion: A randomized trial. *Pediatrics*, *133*(4), e835–e842. https://doi.org/10.1542/peds.2013-2365

Pourebrahim-Alamdari, P., Mehrabi, E., Nourizadeh, R., Esmaeilpour, K., Mousavi, S., & Hakimi, S. (2022). The effect of face-to-face and phone call motivational interviewing on cervical cancer screening. *Cancer Nursing*, *45*(6), E897–E902. https://doi.org/10.1097/ncc.0000000000001089

Resnicow, K., Delacroix, E., Sonneville, K. R., Considine, S., Grundmeier, R. W., Shu, D., Faerber, J. A., Fiks, A. G., Steffes, J., Harris, D., Woo, H., Proctor, T., Wright, M. E., Shone, L. P., Barlow, S. E., Wasserman, R. C., Siegel, R., & Stockwell, M. S. (2024). Outcome of bmi2+: Motivational interviewing to reduce BMI through primary care AAP PROS practices. *Pediatrics*, *153*(2). https://doi.org/10.1542/peds.2023-062462

Ridner, S. L., Ostapchuk, M., Cloud, R. N., Myers, J., Jorayeva, A., & Ling, J. (2014). Using motivational interviewing for smoking cessation in primary care. *Southern Medical Journal*, *107*(5), 314–319. https://doi.org/10.1097/smj.0000000000000106

Rosen, H. (2014). Is obesity a disease or a behavior abnormality? Did the AMA get it right? *Missouri Medicine*, *111*(2), 104–108. https://pmc.ncbi.nlm.nih.gov/articles/PMC6179496/

The Truth About Vaccines. (2025). *How the vaccine schedule in the U.S. has evolved.* https://go.thetruthaboutvaccines.com/vaccine-schedule/?a_bid=96923f6a%26a_aid=5903de82cac79

U.S. Department of Health and Human Services. (2024). *Physical activity guidelines for Americans* (2nd ed.). https://odphp.health.gov/sites/default/files/2019-09/Physical_Activity_Guidelines_2nd_edition.pdf

Wahab, S., Menon, U., & Szalacha, L. A. (2008). Motivational interviewing and colorectal cancer screening: A peek from the inside out. *Patient Education and Counseling*, *72*(2), 210–217. https://doi.org/10.1016/j.pec.2008.03.023

Woolford, S. J., Resnicow, K., Davis, M. M., Nichols, L. P., Wasserman, R. C., Harris, D., Gebremariam, A., Shone, L., Fiks, A. G., & Chang, T. (2022). Cost-effectiveness of a motivational interviewing obesity intervention versus usual care in pediatric primary care offices. *Obesity*, *30*(11), 2265–2274. https://doi.org/10.1002/oby.23560

Chapter 8

Motivational Interviewing Training

Part 1

Training and development: The best development programmes change the way people see themselves.

—John Bright

In this chapter we will explore what basic training in MI looks like, being mindful that it is only through persistent practice in real-life scenarios that true mastery is ever achieved. As you are working through these exercises, ask yourself "Which type of nurse/provider do I want to look like? Which method feels right to me?" Also, understand that just learning about MI is not enough. It will take time, practice, and feedback to master it. One excellent resource for training is the Motivational Interviewing Network of Trainers (MINT), which has multiple training modules open to the public (motivational-interviewing.org/), some of which have been adapted here for the health care profession.[1]

OBJECTIVES

- Students will be able to identify key MI techniques.
- Students will be able to analyze patient-nurse/NP interactions.

1. Exercises and tables in this chapter are adapted from Motivational Interviewing Network of Trainers, *Selections from Motivational Interviewing: Training New Trainers Manual*, pp. 33, 35, 39. Copyright © 2014 by Motivational Interviewing Network of Trainers (CC BY-SA 4.0) at https://www.motivationalinterviewing.org/sites/default/files/tnt_manual_2014_d10_20150205.pdf.

- Students will be able to apply MI techniques in clinical scenarios.
- Students will be able to reflect on personal communication techniques and the impact these have on patients.

Pretraining Quiz

1. What is the primary goal of MI in a health care setting?
    a. To provide direct instructions to patients
    b. To enhance patient motivation and facilitate behavior change
    c. To diagnose medical conditions
    d. To enforce compliance with treatment plans
2. Which of the following best describes the spirit of motivational interviewing?
    a. Confrontational and directive
    b. Collaborative and empathetic
    c. Authoritative and prescriptive
    d. Passive and indifferent
3. What technique is used in MI to reflect back what a patient has said?
    a. Summarizing
    b. Directing
    c. Reflective listening
    d. Questioning
4. How should a nurse respond if a patient expresses resistance to change during a motivational interviewing session?
    a. Ignore the resistance and continue with the plan.
    b. Confront the patient about their lack of motivation.
    c. Explore the reasons behind the resistance and validate the patient's feelings.
    d. Dismiss the patient's concerns as unimportant.
5. Which of the following is *not* a principle of MI?
    a. Autonomy
    b. Collaboration
    c. Judgment
    d. Evocation

Answer Key:

1. b. To enhance patient motivation and facilitate behavior change
2. b. Collaborative and empathetic
3. c. Reflective listening
4. c. Explore the reasons behind the resistance and validate the patient's feelings.
5. c. Judgment

Exercises

Compare and Contrast

For this first exercise, compare both case studies. One reflects the paternalistic/ expert approach, and the other reflects an MI approach. Pay close attention to how each scenario makes you feel.

- Assignment: Write a paper that compares both methods.
- Background: Debby is a female in her 30s with a 7-day history of sinus drainage, facial pain, and headache. Since her last visit she has gained 10 pounds, putting her BMI in the obese category. NP Smith is her primary care provider.

Expert approach:

> *NP Smith* (Looking at the computer, not making any eye contact): "Hello, Debby. What brings you in today?"
>
> *Debby:* "I have had a headache with sinus drainage going on now for a week. Today my face started hurting and I thought I should come in."
>
> *NP Smith* (interrupts her while still looking at the chart): "I understand. But before we get into that, I've noticed your weight has really taken a jump since the last time you were here?"
>
> *Debby* (surprised, shifting uncomfortably): "Well, I have been eating out too much lately, but today I am here because of my sinus infection."
>
> *NP Smith* (sighing): "I totally understand, and we will address that, don't you worry. But this kind of weight gain can have significant impacts on your overall health. I am worried! Weight gain is the leading cause of diabetes. Have you considered joining a weight loss program or talking to a dietician? It could really help you get back on track."

Debby: "I guess … I just want to know if I need antibiotics or something for this."

NP Smith (does a brief physical exam and then resumes charting): "Honestly, losing weight should be your top priority. I'll give you a prescription for some antibiotics for your sinus infection, but I would recommend you start to exercise regularly and watch your portion sizes, cut back on eating out, and incorporate more fruits and vegetables into your diet. I would like to see you back in a month to see how you are doing."

Debby (voice trembling): "Okay …"

NP Smith (handing her a generic pamphlet): "Here is some information on eating healthier and exercise. If this doesn't work maybe we can talk about weight loss medication."

Debby (quietly): "Thank you."

NP Smith (already turning to the computer): "Take care."

- What are your initial reactions to the provider's comments about the patient's weight? Why do you think you feel that way?
- Do you feel the provider's comments were appropriate for this visit?
- What could the provider have done differently to create a more supportive and respectful environment?
- How do you feel the patient felt during this visit?

MI approach:

NP Smith: "Hi, Debby! It's great to see you today. I understand you have had some issues with your sinuses this past week?"

Debby: "I've been really tired this past week, and my nose would not quit running. Today my face started to hurt, and I thought it was best to come it. I am so tired of being tired!"

NP Smith: "It sounds like this infection has really taken you down and you sound frustrated! Is there anything else that has been bothering you or affecting your life?"

Debby: "Well, since I have been sick all week, I have missed Timmy's baseball games and I feel awful about that. But to tell you the truth I have also gained some weight, and that makes going to the games even harder. It gets so hot, and I have noticed I get short of breath now walking across the field. I want to lose these extra pounds, but that seems impossible!"

NP Smith: "It sounds like you feel stuck. Part of you wants to be active with your kids and lose some weight, but the other part says it's too hard. What do you think is the biggest barrier for you right now?"

Debby: "I don't know. I guess I just don't know where to start. It feels so overwhelming. I must work, and then we have a full baseball schedule every night of the week during the summer so that leaves no time to cook at home. Take out just seems easier, but then I get fat!"

NP Smith: "That's completely understandable. Change can feel overwhelming, especially when there are multiple things on your plate like you have just described. What would be one small step you could take to improve how you eat? What's one thing you feel you could manage right now?"

Debby: "Maybe I could investigate those healthy meals that are already prepped for you. At least during the summer?"

NP Smith: "That's a fantastic idea! I hear some of them are good, and they are perfectly proportioned. How do you feel about setting that as a goal for this week?"

Debby: "Yeah, it feels doable."

NP Smith: "Great! I'm proud of you for taking this step. Let's not forget why you came in and get you some medicines for that sinus infection."

Debby: "That sounds good. I do want to feel better."

NP Smith: "Absolutely! I will send your prescription to the pharmacy and remember, I'm here to support you with your weight loss goals too. We can check in on your progress on our next visit. You're doing an amazing job by taking charge of your health!"

Examine each interaction and look at the differences. Give specific examples of how they are different and be prepared to discuss this in class (MINT, 2015).

Table 8.1 Expert verses MI

	Expert Approach	MI Approach
Provider's approach		
Focus of conversation		
Communication style		
Emotional support		
Patient involvement		
Addressing sensitive topics		
Nonverbal communication		
Outcome of the visit		

Twelve Roadblocks to Listening

Thomas Gordon was a prominent psychologist who studied under Carl Rogers. His contributions to the field involved communication and interpersonal relationships, particularly in the field of counseling. Gordon is noted for the following 12 roadblocks to effective listening, otherwise known as the Gordon model. Gordon notes that these reactions stem from wanting to help someone in distress but have the opposite effect. These roadblocks will often lead down the path to ineffective communication instead of fostering the supportive environment that one wants. This is particularly true in the patient-nurse/NP relationship. Health care workers are drawn to this field because they genuinely want to help their patients. You can see how easy it is to fall into the trap of using one of the 12 roadblocks inadvertently:

1. Ordering, directing, or commanding
2. Warning or threatening
3. Giving advice, making suggestions and/or offering solutions
4. Persuading (with logic)
5. Moralizing/preaching/telling

6. Judging/criticizing/disagreeing/blaming
7. Agreeing/approving/praising
8. Shaming, ridiculing, labelling, name-calling
9. Interpreting or analyzing
10. Reassuring, sympathizing, consoling
11. Questioning or probing
12. Withdrawing distracting, humoring, changing the subject (Melnyck, 2019)

This activity is designed to help you pay more attention to these roadblocks by noting them. In the following dialogue, pay attention to what they are saying and how the nurse blocks the conversation with one of the 12 roadblocks and make a note of it for discussion later.

> *Patient:* "I am so anxious. I can't get to sleep. I wish the test results would just come back. I don't know what to do."
>
> *Nurse* (roadblock: reassuring): "Don't worry until you have something to worry about. I'm sure everything will turn out fine. You'll see; it's probably nothing."
>
> *Patient:* "But I can't stop thinking about it no matter what I do. What if it is something serious? How will I tell my husband or my kids? I feel like I'm losing my mind."
>
> *Nurse* (roadblock: advising): "Well, you just try to relax. Maybe try meditating or watching a little TV to get your mind off things. That always helps me when I'm stressed."
>
> *Patient:* "I've tried that, all of that. Nothing seems to work. I feel like I'm stuck in this cycle of worry and can't make it stop."
>
> *Nurse* (roadblock: judging): "You're probably overthinking it. You shouldn't let yourself get so worked up over something that hasn't even happened yet."
>
> *Patient:* "That is easy to say but hard to do. I feel like no one understands how overwhelming this is for me."
>
> *Nurse* (roadblock: ordering): "Don't think like that. Focus on staying positive, and everything will be okay."

Discuss your findings with a partner and then compare your thoughts to the following analysis.

- Reassuring: The nurse's initial response, "Don't worry until you have something to worry about," dismisses the patient's concerns. While the nurse's intention is meant to be comforting, it invalidates the patient's feelings and makes her feel unheard. This prevents further exploration of her anxiety.

- Advising: Suggesting meditation or watching TV without fully understanding the patient's situation comes across as a quick fix. This advice may not be helpful or relevant to the patient's specific needs.
- Judging: Telling the patient they're "overthinking" minimizes their experience and implies that their feelings are irrational, which can make the patient feel judged or misunderstood.
- Ordering: Statements like "Don't think like that" are directive and controlling. They don't empower the patient to explore their emotions or find their own solutions.

In the following example, instead of using roadblocks, the nurse employs MI techniques such as open-ended questions, affirmations, reflections, or summarization to help the patient think through their problem: "I can see how overwhelmed you must be feeling right now. It sounds like all this uncertainty about your tests is making it hard for you to relax. Can you tell me more about what you are thinking?" This approach utilizes MI skills and allows the patient to explore what they are feeling more and with a little more prompting the patient will probably come up with a solution that will work better for them, *and* they will feel the nurse/NP listened to them and acknowledged what they were feeling rather than dismissing their feelings or feeling judged.

Role Play

Practice session 1

Role-play paternalistic/expert assignment: Work in groups of two. One will play the part of the nurse and the other will play the part of the patient.

- Patient: Think of something you are really considering changing in your life.
- Nurse: Your job will be to convince or persuade the patient to make this change. Play the part as if your job depends on them making this change:
    - Explain why the patient needs to make this change.
    - Give three specific benefits from making these changes.
    - Tell them how they could make the change.
    - Explain the importance of making the change.
    - Tell/persuade the person to do it.

If you are unsuccessful at convincing the patient to make the change, try harder for up to two more times, then switch roles.

Discussion or journal reflection:

- How did this encounter made you feel?
- Were you receptive to the advice that you were given?
- Did you feel empowered to make this change?
- Did you need the education that was given?
- How likely will you make the change based on this encounter?

Practice session 2

Role-play MI assignment: Again, you will work in groups of two. One will play the part of the nurse, and the other will play the part of the patient.

- Patient: Consider a change you are considering making in your life.
- Nurse: Your job will be to listen and support the patient in the change they want to make. You cannot try to persuade; do not offer advice, and in the end summarize the encounter to the patient's satisfaction to ensure you heard everything they were saying correctly. In your dialogue ask the following questions:
    - Why would you want to make this change?
    - If you decide to make this change, how might you go about it?
    - What are three reasons for you to make this change?
    - How important is it for you to make this change on a scale of 0–10, with 0 being no confidence and 10 being completely confident?
    - Summarize what you have heard back to the patient and ask if you have left anything out.
    - Ask "So, what do you think you will do?"

  At the end of this encounter switch roles.

  Discussion or journal reflection:

- Discuss how this encounter made you feel.
- Did you feel heard?
- Did you come up with some solutions for your problem?
- Did you feel empowered to make this change?
- How likely will you make the change based on this encounter? (MINT, 2015)

In your journal, write what you have noticed so far about each method:

- Which method (expert/MI) are you leaning towards as a nurse/NP?
- What are your concerns?
- Which method would you prefer as a patient? Why or why not?
- Do you have concerns about time constraints?

Case Study: To Dance or to Wrestle

As you read the following case study, use Table 8.2 (MINT, 2015) to record your thoughts. Try to identify where you think the conversation goes from a 1 (total wrestling) to a 6 (total dancing). When you notice that change, make a note about what is happening in the dialogue.

Scenario: The following is a conversation between NP Emily and her patient, Mr. Carter, a 75-year-old man with a 60-year history of smoking. Mr. Carter has been diagnosed with late-stage chronic obstructive pulmonary disease (COPD) and has been advised to quit smoking to prevent further lung damage.

> *NP Emily:* "Good morning, Mr. Carter. I want to talk to you about your COPD. This disease makes it hard for you to breathe. Your lungs are severely damaged, and smoking is what has caused that damage. It is possible for you to regain a little of the lung function that is not permanently damaged if you stop smoking right away. You really cannot have any more cigarettes."
>
> *Mr. Carter:* "Yeah, I've heard that before. But honestly, I don't think I can quit. I've tried it before, and it just doesn't work for me."
>
> *NP Emily:* "Well, you really need to quit. If you don't, your COPD will only get worse, and you could end up needing oxygen therapy or get lung cancer. This condition can kill you."
>
> *Mr. Carter:* "I get it, but it's just not that easy. Smoking helps me deal with stress, and when I try to quit, I just get more stressed. It's an endless cycle."
>
> *NP Emily* (adjusting her approach):"It sounds like smoking has been a big part of your life, especially when it comes to managing stress. Can you tell me more about what you like about smoking and what it feels like when you try to quit?"
>
> *Mr. Carter:* "Well, when I'm stressed, having a cigarette calms me down. It's like my way of taking a break and relaxing. When I try to quit, I just get more and more anxious."
>
> *NP Emily:* "I see. So, smoking feels like a way to cope with stress and take a moment for yourself. At the same time, you're also dealing with the effects of COPD, which I imagine must be frustrating."

Mr. Carter: "Yeah, it is. I hate feeling short of breath all the time, but I don't know if I can give up smoking. I know that sounds crazy, but it's true."

NP Emily: "It sounds like you're feeling stuck—on one hand, smoking helps you manage stress, but on the other hand withdrawal from nicotine makes you feel more stressed, and smoking is making it harder to breathe affecting your health. What do you think would make it easier for you to consider cutting back or quitting?"

Mr. Carter: "I don't know. I guess if I had something else to ease the feelings of withdrawal, it might be easier. But I've been smoking for so long, it's hard to imagine stopping. I am not sure anything could replace it."

NP Emily: "That makes sense. Quitting something that's been a part of your life for so long can feel overwhelming. What are some things you've tried in the past to manage stress, besides smoking?"

Mr. Carter: "Maybe, I could try the nicotine patches again and see if they help."

NP Emily: "I can help with that."

Table 8.2 **Dialogue**

Wrestling Dancing						**Dialogue**	**MI Technique**
1	2	3	4	5	6	Quote:	Comment on technique used
1	2					Initial phase:	
		3	4			Transitionary phase:	

Wrestling			Dancing			Dialogue	MI Technique
				5	6	Collaborative phase:	

Discuss your results as a class and then compare your thoughts to this analysis.

- **Initial phase: Wrestling (1–2).** At the beginning of the conversation, NP Emily adopts a direct approach, emphasizing the need for Mr. Carter to quit smoking without exploring his feelings or motivations. Statements like "You really cannot have any more cigarettes" create resistance and defensiveness in Mr. Carter. This phase demonstrates the limitations of a directive, expert model, as it fails to engage the patient in meaningful dialogue or address his ambivalence about smoking.
- **Transition phase: Exploring ambivalence (3–4).** NP Emily adjusts her approach by using reflective listening and open-ended questions to explore Mr. Carter's feelings about smoking. For example, she says, "It sounds like you're feeling stuck—on one hand, smoking helps you manage stress, but on the other hand withdrawal from nicotine makes you feel more stressed, and smoking is making it harder to breathe affecting your health. What do you think would make it easier for you to consider cutting back or quitting?" This shift acknowledges Mr. Carter's perspective and begins to explore the tension between the benefits he perceives from smoking and the negative impact it has on his health.
- **Collaborative phase: Dancing (5–6).** In the latter part of the conversation, NP Emily fully transitions to a collaborative approach. She uses open-ended questions, such as "That makes sense. Quitting something that's been a part of your life for so long can feel overwhelming. What are some things you've tried in the past to manage stress, besides smoking?" and engages Mr. Carter in identifying his own solutions. By focusing on small, manageable steps, such as finding alternative ways to manage stress and decreasing symptoms of withdrawal, NP Emily empowers Mr. Carter to take ownership of the change process.

    - Discuss or reflect on as a class other situations you have either worked with a patient or been a patient, and how a visit can feel like a struggle or wrestling match verses like a dance.
    - What can we learn from these types of encounters?

Case Study: Transtheoretical Stages of Change Model

Being able to recognize what stage of change a person is in is important for you to know which approach to take. As you read the dialogue, identify which stages of change Mrs. Taylor is in at different points of the conversation using the transtheoretical stages of change model. Use the scale provided to rate her readiness to change. Record your observations in Table 8.3 (MINT, 2015).

- Stage 1: Precontemplation (not considering change)
- Stages 2–3: Contemplations (thinking about change but not ready to act)
- Stages 4–5: Preparation (planning for change)
- Stage 6: Action (actively making changes)
- Stage 7: Maintenance (sustaining changes over time)

NP: "Good morning, Ms. Taylor. How are you feeling today?"

Mrs. Taylor: "I'm okay, I guess. Just here for my yearly physical. I know I need to lose weight, but honestly, I'm not sure it's something I can do right now. I've tried before, and it never works."

NP: "It sounds like you're feeling a bit discouraged about past attempts. Can you tell me more about what happened when you tried to lose weight before?"

Mrs. Taylor: "Well, I tried a couple of diets, but I always ended up quitting after a few weeks. It's just so hard to stick to it, especially with my busy schedule."

NP: "I hear you. Life can get busy, and making changes can feel overwhelming. What do you think would make it easier for you to stick with a plan this time?"

Mrs. Taylor: "I don't know. Maybe if I had more time or if I didn't have to cook separate meals for my family. It's just hard to balance everything."

NP: "That makes sense. It sounds like time and family responsibilities are big challenges for you. What would you say are the benefits of losing weight, though, if you were able to make it work?"

Mrs. Taylor: "Well, I know it would help me feel better. I get tired a lot, and I don't want to end up with diabetes like my mom."

NP: "So, you're concerned about your health and want to avoid diabetes. That's an important goal. What's one small step you think you could take to start moving in that direction?"

Mrs. Taylor: "Maybe I could try walking a little more. I used to enjoy walking in the evenings, but I haven't done it in a while."

NP: "That's a great idea! Walking is a simple way to get started, and it doesn't require a lot of extra time. How many days a week do you think you could fit in a short walk?"

Mrs. Taylor: "I think I could start with 2 or 3 days a week. I could probably do 20 minutes after dinner."

NP: "That sounds like a solid plan. Starting small is a great way to build momentum. How about we check in next time to see how it's going and talk about other steps you might want to take?"

Mrs. Taylor: "Okay, that sounds good. I think I can try that."

Table 8.3 **Stages of Change**

Stage	Dialogue	MI Technique
Precontemplation		
Contemplation		
Preparation		
Action		

Example analysis:

- Stage 1: Precontemplation (rating: 1)

  - Dialogue: "I know I need to lose weight, but honestly, I'm not sure it's something I can do right now."
  - What's happening: Mrs. Taylor is not ready to act and feels discouraged due to past failures. She is focused on barriers rather than benefits.
  - Prompt for change: The NP uses reflective listening to validate her feelings and asks open-ended questions to explore her past experiences.

- Stage 2: Contemplation (rating: 3)

  - Dialogue: "Maybe if I had more time or if I didn't have to cook separate meals for my family."
  - What's happening: Mrs. Taylor begins to consider what might make change possible, showing ambivalence. She is weighing the pros and cons of making a change.
  - Prompt for change: The NP explores ambivalence by exploring the benefits of losing weight, helping Mrs. Taylor connect her health concerns to her motivation.

- Stage 3: Preparation (rating: 5)

  - Dialogue: "Maybe I could try walking a little more. I used to enjoy walking in the evenings, but I haven't done it in a while."
  - What's happening: Mrs. Taylor starts to identify a specific, manageable action she could take. She is moving from thinking about change to planning for it.
  - Prompt for change: The NP uses affirmation to reinforce her idea and asks a specific question to help her create a realistic plan.

- Stage 4: Action (rating: 6)

  - Dialogue: "I think I could start with 2 or 3 days a week. I could probably do 20 minutes after dinner."
  - What's happening: Mrs. Taylor commits to a concrete plan and is ready to act.
  - Prompt for change: The NP supports her self-efficacy by emphasizing the importance of starting small and offering to follow up.

Reflection questions:

- What techniques did the NP use to help Ms. Taylor move through the stages of change?
- How did the NP support Ms. Taylor's autonomy and self-efficacy?
- What could the NP do on future visits to help Ms. Taylor maintain her progress?

Case Study: OARS Technique

We have talked about using the OARS technique in previous chapters, but now it is time to practice it. Read the following dialogue and listen to each time the nurse uses each of the OARS responses. As you read them, record your impressions in Table 8.4 (MINT, 2015). Make a note of the example used.

- Open ended: "Tell me more about …"
- Affirmation: "You have been successful in …"
- Reflective listening: "It sounds like …"
- Summary: "What we talked about today included …"

> *NP:* "Hi, Mel! It's good to see you today. How have you been feeling lately?"
>
> *Mel:* "Oh, I have been fine. I feel good, just here to get my diabetes checked."
>
> *NP:* "We can certainly do that. Has anything else been a problem?"
>
> *Mel:* "Julie left for college. She was our last kid, and I am retiring. Find myself drinking a bit more than I used to. My wife thinks it's becoming a problem."
>
> *NP:* "What are your thoughts on that?"
>
> *Mel:* "Well, drinking helps me unwind, but I know it is keeping my sugar diabetes high."
>
> *NP:* "I appreciate you sharing that with me. It sounds like on the one hand you want to stop drinking because you know it is making your diabetes worse, but on the other hand it helps you to unwind."
>
> *Mel:* "Exactly, I just don't want it to get out of control."
>
> *NP:* "It's great that you're aware of your feelings and want to address them. Let's summarize what we've talked about: You've been drinking more lately since Julie left for college, and you have retired. While it helps you unwind, you're worried about it becoming a problem. Does that sound right?"
>
> *Mel:* "Yes, that's exactly it."

Table 8.4 OARS

Nurse/NP Response	Good Dialogue
Open-ended questions	
Affirmation	
Reflection	
Summary	

Example analysis:

- Open-ended questions
  - Example: "Has anything else been a problem?"
  - Purpose: This question invites Mel to elaborate on his situation, providing the NP with valuable insight into his drinking habits and stressors.
- Affirmation
  - Example: "I appreciate you sharing that with me."
  - Purpose: This statement acknowledges Mel's feelings and reinforces his openness, helping to build trust and rapport.
- Reflective listening
  - Example: "It sounds like on the one hand you want to stop drinking because you know it is making your diabetes worse, but on the other hand, it helps you to unwind."
  - Purpose: This reflection validates Mel's internal conflict and encourages him to explore his feelings further.
- Summarizing

- Example: "It's great that you're aware of your feelings and want to address them. Let's summarize what we've talked about: You've been drinking more lately since Julie left for college, and you have retired. While it helps you unwind, you're worried about it becoming a problem. Does that sound right?"
- Purpose: The summary helps organize the conversation, ensures mutual understanding, and sets the stage for collaborative planning.

Post-training Quiz

1. What is the primary goal of MI?
   a. To provide direct advice to patients
   b. To enhance patient motivation and facilitate behavior change
   c. To diagnose medical conditions
   d. To enforce compliance with treatment plans
2. Which of the following is an example of an open-ended question?
   a. "Are you feeling better today?"
   b. "What changes have you considered making to improve your health?"
   c. "Do you understand the treatment plan?"
   d. "Is your pain manageable?"
3. What does the "A" in the OARS technique stand for?
   a. Advice
   b. Acknowledgment
   c. Affirmation
   d. Assessment
4. Which of the following is a roadblock to effective listening according to Thomas Gordon?
   a. Reflective listening
   b. Ordering or directing
   c. Summarizing
   d. Empathy
5. In the context of MI, what does reflective listening involve?
   a. Providing solutions to the patient's problems
   b. Repeating what the patient says verbatim
   c. Paraphrasing or summarizing the patient's feelings and thoughts
   d. Asking rapid-fire questions to gather information

6. What is the significance of exploring ambivalence in a patient's behavior?
    a. It helps the provider judge the patient's readiness for change
    b. It allows the patient to articulate their conflicting feelings about change
    c. It encourages the provider to give more advice
    d. It simplifies the conversation
7. Which stage of change involves a patient actively planning to make a change?
    a. Precontemplation
    b. Contemplation
    c. Preparation
    d. Action
8. What is an effective way to support a patient's autonomy during a conversation?
    a. By telling them what they should do
    b. By asking for their input and preferences
    c. By providing unsolicited advice
    d. By minimizing their concerns
9. How can summarizing be beneficial in a patient-provider conversation?
    a. It allows the provider to dominate the conversation
    b. It helps clarify and reinforce the main points discussed
    c. It provides an opportunity to give advice
    d. It ends the conversation quickly
10. What is the impact of using affirmations in a health care setting?
    a. They can make patients feel judged
    b. They help build rapport and encourage patient engagement
    c. They are unnecessary in clinical conversations
    d. They distract from the main issues

Answer Key:

1. b. To enhance patient motivation and facilitate behavior change
2. b. "What changes have you considered making to improve your health?"
3. c. Affirmation
4. b. Ordering or directing
5. c. Paraphrasing or summarizing the patient's feelings and thoughts
6. b. It allows the patient to articulate their conflicting feelings about change
7. c. Preparation
8. b. By asking for their input and preferences

9. b. It helps clarify and reinforce the main points discussed
10. b. They help build rapport and encourage patient engagement

References

Melnyck, R. (2019, July 24). *12 Communication roadblocks: Beware of these dirty dozen.* Prime Your Pump. https://primeyourpump.com/2019/07/24/12-communication-roadblocks/

Motivational Interviewing Network of Trainers. (2015). *Motivational interviewing training new trainers model.* https://www.motivationalinterviewing.org/sites/default/files/tnt_manual_2014_d10_20150205.pdf

Chapter 9

Motivational Interviewing Training

Part 2

Practice isn't the thing you do once you're good. It's the thing you do that makes you good.

—Malcolm Gladwell

Building on the foundational techniques introduced in the previous chapter, this chapter will further break down skillful application of MI strategies.[1] Think of this as day 2 of your MI seminar, remembering that while knowledge of MI strategies is essential, skillful application requires ongoing engagement with the method in real-world contexts. Learning MI will require vulnerability on your part as you try out new ways of interacting with patients. As you work through the following exercises, reflect on the type of nurse or provider you aim to become. We know this is not a process with a finish line, so even if you've been a practicing nurse or provider for years, think of ways you want to grow. Which MI strategies come the most easily to you? Which of them already aligns with your current approach to patient communication? Which techniques may require more intentional practice to integrate effectively?

Consider which elements of MI closely reflect your personal values and communication patterns. Remember, competence is not achieved through conceptual understanding alone. It develops over time through repeated practice, self-reflection, and meaningful feedback. You will know what works for you once you apply it to patients see how it impacts them and how it impacts *you*.

1. Exercises and tables in this chapter are adapted from Motivational Interviewing Network of Trainers, Selections from *Motivational Interviewing: Training New Trainers Manual*, pp. 38, 63, 66–67, 77–79, 116–117, 120–121, 202–205. Copyright © 2014 by Motivational Interviewing Network of Trainers (CC BY-SA 4.0) at https://www.motivationalinterviewing.org/sites/default/files/tnt_manual_2014_d10_20150205.pdf.

OBJECTIVES

- Students will be able to identify advanced MI techniques.
- Students will be able to analyze patient-nurse/NP interactions.
- Students will be able to apply MI techniques in clinical scenarios.
- Students will be able to reflect on personal communication styles and the impact this has on patients.

Pretraining Quiz

1. Which of the following is an example of recognizing a client's change talk cue?
   a. "I don't think I have a problem."
   b. "Maybe I could try cutting back a little."
   c. "My friend says I should stop, but I don't care."
   d. "It's just the way I am."
2. When a patient expresses resistance, which MI technique is most appropriate?
   a. Confront the patient directly.
   b. Ignore the resistance.
   c. Roll with the resistance.
   d. Provide unsolicited advice.
3. Which response best demonstrates the MI skill of reflective listening?
   a. "You should really consider quitting."
   b. "Why don't you want to change?"
   c. "It sounds like you're worried about what might happen if you stop."
   d. "Let's make a plan right now."
4. A patient says, "I know I should exercise, but I just don't have time." What is the best MI response?
   a. "You'll need to make time."
   b. "You're feeling overwhelmed by your schedule, but you also see the value in exercising."
   c. "That's just an excuse."
   d. "Let's talk about your diet instead."

Answer Key:

1. b. "Maybe I could try cutting back a little."

2. c. Roll with the resistance.
3. c. "It sounds like you're worried about what might happen if you stop."
4. b. "You're feeling overwhelmed by your schedule, but you also see the value in exercising."

Exercises

Change Talk

It is important for you to be able to identify when you hear change talk. As you read, the following case study use Table 9.1 (Motivational Interviewing Network of Trainers [MINT], 2015) to record your thoughts. Try to identify where you think the conversation goes from a *desire* to change to the *ability* to change to the *reasons* to change to the *need* for change and finally the *commitment* to change.

> *Nurse:* "Hi, Mr. Lee. I understand you've been thinking about your smoking lately. Can you tell me a bit about what's on your mind?"
>
> *Mr. Lee:* "Well, I guess I'd like to quit smoking. I've been thinking about it more these days."
>
> *Nurse:* "It sounds like quitting is something you want. What makes you feel that way?"
>
> *Mr. Lee:* "I just feel tired all the time, and I notice I get out of breath easily. I think I could quit if I really tried."
>
> *Nurse:* "You believe you have what it takes to quit. What are some reasons quitting is important to you?"
>
> *Mr. Lee:* "My kids have been asking me to stop, and I want to be around for them as they grow up. Plus, I know it would help my health."
>
> *Nurse:* "Those sound like powerful reasons. How important is it for you to make this change now?"
>
> *Mr. Lee:* "Honestly, I need to do this soon. My doctor said my lungs aren't in great shape, and I don't want things to get worse."
>
> *Nurse:* "You're seeing that it's necessary to quit. What do you think your next step will be?"
>
> *Mr. Lee:* "I'm going to set a quit date for next month and talk to my doctor about some support options."

Table 9.1 Change Talk

Type of Change Talk	Dialogue Example
Desire to change	
Ability to change	
Reasons to change	
Need to change	
Commitment to change	

- Desire to change: "Well, I guess I'd like to quit smoking. I've been thinking about it more these days." This is a classic example of *desire change talk* as the patient expresses a wish or preference to quit.
- Ability to change: "I just feel tired all the time, and I notice I get out of breath easily. I think I could quit if I really tried." Here the patient expresses *ability change talk*. Specifically, the phrase "I think I could quit if I really tried" reflects the patient's belief in their capacity to change which is very important.
- Reasons to change: "My kids have been asking me to stop, and I want to be around for them as they grow up. Plus, I know it would help my health." This response contains *reasons* change talk. The patient provides meaningful reasons they should make this change.
- Need to change: "Honestly, I need to do this soon. My doctor said my lungs aren't in great shape, and I don't want things to get worse." This is an example of *need* change talk. The patient expresses a sense of urgency or necessity to make this change, including medical reasons and a desire to avoid a negative outcome.

- Commitment to change: "I'm going to set a quit date for next month and talk to my doctor about some support options." This type of *commitment* change talk is very powerful. The patient is not only expressing an intention but has outlined specific steps they will take.

Change talk versus Sustain Talk

Change talk consists of patient statements that reflect a desire, ability, reason, need or commitment to make a positive change. Sustain talk consists of patient statements that resist change. Using Table 9.2, place a C for *change talk*, S for *sustain talk*, and O for *other talk* to identify the following statements (MINT, 2015).

Table 9.2 Change or Sustain

Statement	**Change/Sustain/Other Talk**
"Yes, I believe I can remember to take my medicine."	
"I know I'd feel better if I started exercising more."	
"I've tried losing weight before; it just doesn't work for me."	
"My friend recently joined a gym and seemed to like it."	
"Maybe I could start by just walking more each day."	
"I'm not sure if I'm ready to quit smoking right now."	
"Honestly, I don't have the time to work out."	
"I should schedule my check up next month"	
"If my husband can lose weight, I can too."	
"My friend lost a lot of weight taking a GLP-1."	
"I don't think I could give up my nightly glass of wine."	

Statement	Change/Sustain/Other Talk
"Sometimes I feel stressed, but I don't know what to do."	

Answer Key: C, C, S, O, C, S, S, O, C, O, S, S, O

Evoking Change Talk

Practice identifying change talk in mixed patient statements and respond with reflections that will emphasize and amplify the change talk to help increase the client motivation.

1. Read each patient's statement carefully. Notice how the statements contain both sustain talk (reasons to stay the same) and change talk (reasons or desires to change).
2. Underline or highlight the change talk.
3. Write a reflective statement that focuses only on the change talk part, intentionally ignoring the sustain talk or resistance.
4. Share your reflections with a partner or group or in your reflection journal.

Patient: "I am 78 years old, and this medication metformin is ruining what life and pleasure I have left. I can't even leave the house because I am constantly in the bathroom. I know the doctor said there is a good chance it will help my diabetes, but I don't think the side effects are worth it."

- Identify the change talk: "I know it's supposed to help my diabetes."
- Write a reflection focusing on the change talk: "It's pretty clear that the doctor wants you to continue."

Patient: "The material the clinic gave me for my high blood pressure said I should avoid processed food or else read the labels. I'm so busy I barely have time to eat, let alone shop, analyze my groceries, and spend half the night in the kitchen. These people do not live in the real world."

- Identify the change talk.
- Write a reflection focusing on the change talk.

Patient: "Is it such a crime that I want to enjoy life while I'm still young? Once I'm tied into work, paying the bills, kids and all that I can scale things back."

- Identify the change talk.
- Write a reflection focusing on the change talk.

Patient: "It is so frustrating that the minute you get pregnant everyone expects you to be perfect! I am so stressed out; it can't be good for the baby. I'm only having a few cigarettes a day, and my partner is totally on my case about it.

- Identify the change talk.
- Write a reflection focusing on the change talk.

Reflective practice questions:

- How easy or difficult was it to identify the change talk in each statement?
- How did focusing your reflection on the change talk affect the tone or direction of your response?
- What challenges did you face in ignoring the sustain talk or resistance?
- How might this skill help you in real clinical conversations? (MINT, 2015)

Expressing Compassion

In small groups, spend 20 minutes discussing the following:

- What is compassion?
- How is it effectively expressed?
- What are some reasons to express compassion?
- What makes it easy to express?
- What makes it difficult to express?
- How is it different than empathy?

Discuss findings as a whole class or reflect on them in your journal:

1. Write a description of an actual patient for whom it was easy to express compassion.
2. Write a description of an actual patient for whom it was *not* easy to express compassion.

Discuss these scenarios. Working together, answer the following:

- Identify at least five strengths for a patient.
- Develop at least five affirmations for this patient, including the expression of appreciation/understanding of any difficulties they face.
- Develop at least five simple reflections to express understanding of what the client says.
- Discuss insights learned through this activity as a group. (MINT, 2015)

Compassion and the Spirit of MI

Think of a time you had a difficult or challenging patient. Read the dialogue between a provider and a patient who would be challenging. Take notes to see when you hear an element of MI being used—and the effect it has on the session by using Table 9.3 (MINT, 2015).

> *Patient:* "Honestly, the only reason I'm here is because my wife made me come. I don't really think I need to be here, and I doubt you—or anyone else—can really understand what it's like to be me. This isn't something I want to do."
>
> *Provider:* "Thank you for being honest with me. It sounds like you're feeling a lot of pressure right now and maybe are even a bit frustrated about being here when it wasn't really your choice."
>
> *Patient:* "Yeah, that's exactly it. I just want everyone to leave me alone about my drinking. They don't get it."
>
> *Provider:* "It seems like people around you are worried, but for you drinking is something that's personal, and maybe even a way you cope with things. Is that right?"
>
> *Patient:* "I guess so. I mean, it helps me deal with stress. Work's been rough, and drinking is just … part of how I get through the day."
>
> *Provider:* "That makes sense. You've found something that helps you manage stress, even if others don't see it that way. I'm not here to judge or tell you what to do. My role is to listen and understand your perspective. If you decide you want to talk about your drinking, or if there's anything you'd like to change, I'm here to support you in whatever way you choose."
>
> Patient: "I appreciate that. I just don't want to be lectured to."
>
> *Provider:* "Absolutely. This is your life, and any decisions about it are yours to make. If it's okay with you, maybe we can talk a bit about what you like about drinking, and if there's anything about it that concerns you—even just a little. But only if you feel comfortable."
>
> *Patient:* "Well … I do like how it helps me relax, but I guess sometimes I worry about how much I'm drinking. My wife says I'm not the same person when I've had too much."
>
> *Provider:* "That sounds tough—on both you and your wife. It's normal to have mixed feelings about something that's both helpful and causing some problems. If you ever want to explore those

feelings more, I'm here to help you figure out what's best for you, at your own pace."

Table 9.3 Elements of MI

Element of MI	Example	Effect on the Session

Explore your feelings by answering the following questions in a journal:

- How are you feeling about this appointment?
- What are your thoughts about this patient?
- What are your expectations for the outcome?
- How do you feel about the patient's motivation or ability to change?
- How do you feel regarding his potential?
- What motivations, strengths, or resources do you think he has to draw upon?
- Which element of the SPIRIT of MI (partnership, acceptance, compassion, and evocation) would you apply to this situation?

To give you a greater understanding of this patient, listen to *The Lost Boy* by Greg Holden: youtube.com/watch?v=rNhToEXdDCQ. Reconsider the same questions.

- How are you feeling about this appointment?
- What are your thoughts about this patient?
- What are your expectations for the outcome?
- How do you feel about the patient's motivation or ability to change?
- How do you feel regarding his potential?

- What motivations, strengths, or resources do you think he has to draw upon?
- Which element of the SPIRIT of MI (partnership, acceptance, compassion, and evocation) would you apply to this situation?
- Did your answers change? Is so, what influenced them? (MINT, 2015)

Listening

Practice listening and comprehension skills.

> *NP:* "Good morning, Mr. Johnson. How have you been feeling since your last appointment?"
>
> *Patient:* "Honestly, I've been struggling a bit. I get tired quickly and sometimes feel overwhelmed with all the changes I'm supposed to make."
>
> *NP:* "That sounds really challenging. What changes have been the hardest for you to manage?"
>
> *Patient:* "Mostly diet and exercise. I want to do better, but it's tough to find motivation and time."
>
> *NP:* "It's understandable to feel that way. What do you think might help you stay motivated?"
>
> *Patient:* "Maybe if I had some support or a plan that fits my schedule better."
>
> *NP:* "That's a great insight. We can work together to create a plan that suits you. How about we start with small steps?"

Write a short journal entry answering these questions:

- What do you think the patient is feeling and experiencing?
- What challenges are the patient facing?
- How does the NP respond to the patient's concerns?
- What suggestions or ideas does the patient have for overcoming difficulties?
- What is the NP's approach to helping the patient?

After journaling, review the dialogue again and compare your answers:

- Did you accurately capture the patient's feelings and challenges?
- How well did you notice the NP's empathetic and supportive responses?
- Were you able to identify the collaborative nature of the NPs approach?

- What did you learn about active listening from this exercise?

Using the journal reflections write a short paper describing the following three elements:

- Analyzes the patient's emotional and motivational state.
- Evaluates the NP's communication techniques (e.g., empathy, open-ended questions).
- Suggests ways the NP could further support the patient's behavior change (MINT, 2015).

How Well Do You Listen?

Evaluate communication skills and reflective practice by working in pairs: one nurse and one patient. The student playing the patient will talk for 90 seconds of a habit, behavior, dilemma or situation that they are thinking about changing. The student playing the nurse is tasked with active listening without saying anything or asking any questions. They must then give a summary to the patient's satisfaction. If they leave anything out, they must listen again until the patient is satisfied; they were heard correctly. Then change roles: The student playing the patient will talk for 90 seconds of a habit, behavior, dilemma or situation that they are thinking about changing. The student playing the nurse is tasked with active listening without saying anything or asking any questions. They must give a summary to the patient's satisfaction. If they leave anything out, they must listen again until the patient is satisfied; they were heard correctly. This time the summary may include what the nurse thinks is the underlying meaning, feeling, or dilemma in the story they've heard.

- What is the difference between the two types of summaries? Which one was more difficult? Why?
- How was it for the patient?
- How was it for the nurse? (MINT, 2015)

Practicing Rolling With Resistance

Develop skills in recognizing patient resistance and responding by "rolling with resistance" using reflective listening and other MI techniques.

- Read the following patient statements carefully. Each statement contains some form of resistance (sustain talk or discord).
- Write down how you would respond to each statement using the spirit of MI and the rolling with resistance approach.
    - Avoid arguing, persuading, or correcting.
    - Use reflective listening (simple, amplified, or double-sided reflections).
    - Emphasize client autonomy and avoid pushing for change.

    - Consider shifting focus or validating the client's perspective.
- After writing your response, reflect on why you chose that approach and how it might help maintain rapport and open the door for future change talk.

Statement 1: *"I don't have a problem with drinking. You can tell me all you want, but I'm not going to stop drinking with my friends."*

Response: *"It sounds like drinking with your friends is an important part of your life, and you don't see it as a problem right now."*

Statement 2: *"Alcoholic Anonymous won't help me. I've tried it before and nothing changed."*

Response:

Statement 3: *"You don't understand what it's like for me. Nobody does."*

Response:

Statement 4: *"Diets do not work for me. I have tried them and I might lose some weight but then I gain it all back again. It is no use."*

Response:

Reflection questions:

- How did your response avoid confrontation or persuasion?
- In what ways did your response acknowledge and validate the client's feelings or perspective?
- How might your response encourage the client to continue talking rather than shutting down?
- What challenges did you face in resisting the urge to "correct" or "convince" the client? (MINT, 2015)

Developing the Change Plan

Imagine you are a health care provider working with a client who has expressed some motivation to change a behavior (smoking, drinking, weight loss, illicit drugs, etc.) Your goal is to help the client develop a change plan collaboratively. Write a dialogue (about 8–10 lines) in which you help a patient create a plan or do a role-play between two students; one plays the part of the patient and one the part of the NP.

- Asking open-ended, evocative questions to explore what the client wants to do next.
- Reflect the client's statements to deepen their thinking.
- Affirm the client's autonomy and strengths.
- Avoid giving any direct advice, instructions, or expert opinions.
- Make sure you use reflections that capture both sides of ambivalence if present.
- Be sure to emphasize the client's control over the plan.

Example questions:

- What steps do you think you might take?
- How would you like to approach this?
- What has worked for you in the past?
- What feels doable to you right now?

Avoid the Traps

Be able to recognize when you are slipping back into the paternalistic or expert model.

MI, correct approach:

> *NP:* "You've shared some great reasons for wanting to change. What do you think would be a good first step for you?"
>
> *Patient:*"Maybe I could try cutting back a little this week."
>
> *NP:* "Cutting back a bit sounds like a manageable start. What might that look like for you day-to-day?"
>
> *Patient:* "I could skip my usual after-dinner cigarette a few times."
>
> *NP:* "That sounds like a concrete plan. Do you feel ready to try? How confident do you feel about doing that?"
>
> *Patient:* "I think I can do it, but I'm a little worried about cravings."
>
> *NP:* "It's understandable to feel some worry. What might help you handle those cravings if they come up?"
>
> *Patient:* "Maybe I could go for a walk or call a friend."
>
> *NP:* "Those are great strategies you've thought of. You're really taking charge of this plan."

It is easy to forget our MI skills at this stage of the game. To illustrate, read the following example when the NP does very good in the beginning but then slips back into the paternalistic/expert mode at the end. Note where this happens and how this makes you feel.

MI, incorrect method, slipped back into expert pattern:

> *NP:* "Hi, Mr. Carter. I appreciate you coming in today. Can you tell me a little about what brings you here and what's been on your mind regarding your drinking?"
>
> *Patient:* "Honestly, I'm not sure I'm ready to quit, but I have been feeling more tired lately, and my wife's been worried."
>
> *NP:* "It sounds like you're feeling some pressure, but you've also noticed some changes in your health. What are some things you like about drinking, and what are some things you're less happy about?"
>
> *Patient:* "Well, I like how it helps me relax after work, but I don't like how groggy I feel in the mornings. And I guess I'm starting to worry about my blood pressure."
>
> *NP:* "That makes sense. On one hand, it helps you unwind, but on the other, you're noticing some health effects that concern you. What do you think would be a good next step for you?"
>
> *Patient:* "I'm not sure. Maybe I could try cutting back a little, but I don't know if I can stop completely."
>
> *NP:* "Cutting back is a good idea, but based on your health and what we know about alcohol's effects, the best thing for you would be to stop drinking altogether. I recommend you enroll in our outpatient program starting next week. I'll set you up with an appointment, and you'll need to attend three sessions a week. This is the most effective way to address your concerns and improve your health."
>
> *Patient:* "Oh … okay. I guess if you think that's best."

Discuss in class the difference between these two scenarios or write a paper and answer the following questions:

- How did the NP approach differ in each scenario?
- In which scenario did the patient seem more engaged?

- How did the NP's language and tone influence the patients' motivation or resistance in each scenario?
- What role did empathy and respect for patient autonomy play in each interaction?
- Identify moments when the provider either evoked or suppressed the patients' own reasons for change.
- How did the provider's use of questions differ between the two scenarios?
- What feelings or attitudes might the patient experience in each scenario?
- Reflect on a time when you or someone you know experience a similar interaction. How did the communication style affect the outcome?
- What lessons about the spirit of MI can you draw from comparing these two dialogues?
- How might the provider in the expert-mode scenario shift their approach to better align with MI principles and improve patient engagement? (MINT, 2015)

Change Talk Role-Play and Reflection

Personally experience and identify different types of change talk by role-playing all five types themselves and reflecting on the differences of each. Prepare five statements regarding something you want to change. Then, complete the following statements following the DARN-CAT framework:

- Desire: "I want to ..."
- Ability: "I could ..."
- Reasons: "I have good reasons to ..."
- Need: "I need to ..."
- Commitment: "I will ..."

1. Role-play
    - Think of a change you want to make. Imagine you are the patient and write a statement for each of the five types of change talk (desire, ability, reasons, need, commitment) regarding this change.
    - One student plays the patient and one the NP. Go through the scenario until all five statements have been read, then switch parts.
2. Reflections: Either journal responses or discussion in class
    - How did it feel to say each statement?
    - What did each statement communicate about the motivation or readiness to change?
    - Which statement felt stronger and more decisive?
    - How would you respond differently to each statement as the NP? (MINT, 2015)

Future Practice

Now that you have been through the exercises from both Part 1 and Part 2, write a letter to your future self, from the point of view 5 years from now. Describe what type of nurse or provider you will be and what the interactions will look like between you and your patients. Offer words of encouragement, wisdom, perspective, and hope to your future perspective. Write from the first person (I) to yourself (you) in the present.

Dear Future Me,

Post-Training Quiz

1. Which of the following is *not* one of the four core processes of MI?
    a. Engaging
    b. Focusing
    c. Planning
    d. Diagnosing
2. The spirit of MI includes all the following *except*
    a. Partnership
    b. Acceptance
    c. Confrontation
    d. Compassion
3. Which of the following best describes change talk?
    a. Statements in favor of maintaining the status quo
    b. Statements indicating a desire, ability, reason, or need to change
    c. Statements about other people's problems
    d. Statements that avoid discussing change
4. Rolling with resistance means
    a. arguing with the client
    b. ignoring the client's concerns
    c. accepting and exploring the client's reluctance
    d. forcing the client to change
5. Which is an example of a reflective listening statement?
    a. "You should try harder."
    b. "It sounds like you're feeling frustrated."
    c. "Why did you do that?"
    d. "Let's move on."
6. In MI, "developing discrepancy" refers to
    a. pointing out the client's mistakes.
    b. helping the client see the difference between their goals and current behavior.
    c. ignoring the client's values.
    d. giving direct advice.
7. Which of the following is an open-ended question?
    a. "Do you want to quit?"
    b. "How many drinks do you have per week?"

c. "What are your thoughts about making a change?"
d. "Is this your first attempt?"

8. The acronym OARS stands for

a. open questions, affirmations, reflections, summaries
b. options, actions, results, solutions
c. openings, answers, responses, suggestions
d. objectives, actions, results, summaries

9. Which is an example of sustain talk?

a. "I want to quit smoking."
b. "I don't think I can change right now."
c. "My health is important to me."
d. "I'm ready to try."

10. The primary goal of MI is to

a. convince the client to change.
b. elicit and strengthen the client's own motivation for change.
c. diagnose mental health disorders.
d. provide step-by-step instructions.

11. The four processes of MI are engaging, ____________, evoking, and planning.
12. In MI, the provider's role is to guide rather than _________ the client.
13. ___________listening is a key skill in MI that involves restating or paraphrasing what the client says.
14. The acronym DARN stands for desire, ability, _________ and need.
15. The righting reflex refers to the urge to _________the client's problems.
16. Sort the following MI skills in the correct order of the four processes: engaging, planning, focusing, evoking.
17. Sort the following statements as either change talk or sustain talk:

    - "I want to stop drinking."
    - "I don't think I can quit."
    - "My family would be happier if I changed."
    - "I've tried before and failed."

18. Identify the type of change talk in this statement: "I need to start exercising for my health."
19. Identify the MI principle demonstrated: Provider says, "You're feeling stuck, but you also want things to be different."
20. Identify which OARS skill is being used: Provider says, "That's a great insight—you've shown a lot of strength."

21. Identify the process: Provider helps the client set a quit date and plan for triggers.
22. Identify the MI trap: Provider repeatedly gives advice without asking for permission.
23. Which of the following are components of the spirit of MI? (Select all that apply.)

    a. Partnership
    b. Authority
    c. Acceptance
    d. Compassion

24. Which are examples of affirmations? (Select all that apply.)

    a. "You've worked hard to get this far."
    b. "You never do anything right."
    c. "It took courage to come here today."
    d. "You're always making excuses."

25. Which of the following are open-ended questions? (Select all that apply.)

    a. "What would you like to see different?"
    b. "Do you want to quit?"
    c. "How do you feel about your progress?"
    d. "Is this your first time?"

26. Which are examples of reflective listening? (Select all that apply.)

    a. "It sounds like you're worried about your health."
    b. "Why don't you just stop?"
    c. "You're not sure if you can do this."
    d. "You should try harder."

27. Which of the following are types of change talk? (Select all that apply.)

    a. Desire
    b. Ability
    c. Blame
    d. Need

28. Briefly describe the difference between change talk and sustain talk.
29. Why is it important to avoid the righting reflex in MI?

Answer Key:

1. d. Diagnosing
2. c. Confrontation
3. b. Statements indicating a desire, ability, reason, or need to change

4. c. Accepting and exploring the client's reluctance
5. b. "It sounds like you're feeling frustrated."
6. b. Helping the client see the difference between their goals and current behavior
7. c. "What are your thoughts about making a change?"
8. a. Open questions, affirmations, reflections, summaries
9. b. "I don't think I can change right now."
10. b. Elicit and strengthen the client's own motivation for change
11. Focusing
12. Direct (or tell)
13. Reflective
14. Reasons
15. Fix (or correct)
16. Engaging → focusing → evoking → planning
17.
    - "I want to stop drinking." Change talk
    - "I don't think I can quit." Sustain talk
    - "My family would be happier if I changed." Change talk
    - "I've tried before and failed." Sustain talk
18. Need (expresses necessity to change)
19. Acceptance (MI principle of accepting client's feelings without judgment)
20. Affirmation (recognizing client's strengths)
21. Planning (fourth MI process involving setting goals and strategies)
22. Giving unsolicited advice (MI trap that can cause resistance)
23. Components of MI spirit: a–c
24. Affirmations: a and b
25. Open-ended questions: a and b
26. Reflective listening: a and b
27. Types of change talk: a–c
28. Change talk includes client statements that favor movement toward change (desire, ability, reasons, need, commitment), while sustain talk includes statements that favor maintaining current behavior or rsisting change.
29. "You're feeling frustrated about your drinking, but you also see some benefits to it right now."
30. The righting reflex is the urge to correct or fix the client's problems, which can lead to resistance. Avoiding it helps maintain collaboration, respects client autonomy, and supports intrinsic motivation.

Reference

Motivational Interviewing Network of Trainers. (2015). *Motivational interviewing training new trainers manual.* https://www.motivationalinterviewing.org/sites/default/files/tnt_manual_2014_d10_20150205.pdf

Chapter 10

Cultural Considerations in Motivational Interviewing

Building Bridges in Collaborative Healthcare

You don't see things as they are. You see them as you are.

—Anaïs Nin

While we have created this chapter to address cultural considerations in MI, we do want to stress that culture is not separate or an entity of its own that stands apart from MI. Rather, culture is interwoven into MI so intricately that the two concepts cannot be separated (Lee, 2025). The foundations of MI evolve out of humanistic counseling, which already has at its core the belief that patients are the experts on their own lives and that we are to view the totality of a person and their unique experiences (Rogers, 1951, 1961; Cain, 2010; Miller & Rollnick, 2013; North & Alarik, 2022). Culture is not divorced from the person. Culture lies at the core of personal experience, and MI fosters respectful engagement by acknowledging and valuing this complexity. This means that the spirit of MI already leads into an attitude of cultural awareness, so while we discuss cultural factors in this chapter, you will not have to rework all that you have learned with MI thus far. Rather, you will use the foundational knowledge that we have established to learn how to address cultural factors and support patients in ways that are even stronger and that work with, not against, their cultural background and experiences.

STUDENT OBJECTIVES

- Students will be able to describe the historical and structural roots of healthcare inequities in the United States.
- Students will define key concepts such as cultural competency, cultural humility, and intersectionality.

- Students will identify how cultural factors influence health behaviors and patient-provider interactions.
- Students will learn to apply MI with cultural awareness and responsiveness.
- Students will reflect on personal biases and power dynamics in clinical encounters.
- Students will understand the current research on MI with racially, ethnically, and culturally diverse populations.
- Students will utilize tools and strategies to adapt MI to better support diverse populations.

KEY TERMS AND DEFINITIONS

- **Change talk**: In MI, statements by the patient that indicate motivation for change, including desire, ability, reasons, need, and commitment.
- **Cultural competency**: An earlier approach to intercultural care that focuses on acquiring knowledge about specific cultural groups, often criticized for promoting static and stereotypical understandings.
- **Cultural humility**: A lifelong process of self-reflection and self-critique that acknowledges power imbalances in healthcare and promotes respect, curiosity, and shared learning in the provider-patient relationship.
- **Cultural strengths**: Beliefs, practices, values, and community-based supports rooted in culture that contribute to resilience, healing, and motivation for change.
- **Culturally adapted motivational interviewing (CAMI)**: A framework developed by Christina S. Lee that integrates cultural values, identity, and context into MI practice to enhance engagement, trust, and relevance for diverse populations.
- **Culture**: A dynamic and multifaceted system of beliefs, values, customs, and social behaviors that shape how individuals understand and engage with the world, including their health and healing practices.
- **Ecological validity framework**: A model used to guide the cultural adaptation of interventions.
    - **Context**: The setting in which the intervention is delivered and the manner of its delivery.
    - **Content**: The language, symbols, and materials used to ensure cultural relevance.
    - **Concepts**: The deeper cultural beliefs, values, and worldviews that shape how people understand and respond to the intervention.
- **Evocation**: A core MI process involving drawing out a person's own thoughts, values, and motivations for change rather than imposing external advice.
- **Health disparities**: Preventable differences in health outcomes and access to care experienced

by socially disadvantaged populations.

- **High-context communication**: A communication style in which meaning is conveyed implicitly through context, nonverbal cues, and shared understanding; common in collectivist cultures.
- **Historical trauma**: The cumulative emotional and psychological wounding across generations resulting from massive group trauma experiences such as colonization, slavery, or forced relocation.
- **Implicit bias**: Unconscious attitudes or stereotypes that affect understanding, actions, and decisions in an unintentional manner.
- **Intersectionality**: A framework for understanding how multiple social identities (e.g., race, gender, class, disability) intersect and contribute to unique experiences of oppression and privilege.
- **Low-context communication**: A communication style in which meaning is conveyed explicitly through direct verbal expression; common in individualist cultures.
- **Medical mistrust**: Reluctance or suspicion toward medical systems often rooted in historical exploitation, discrimination, and inequities experienced by marginalized communities.
- **Motivational interviewing (MI)**: A collaborative, person-centered counseling style designed to elicit and strengthen motivation for change by honoring autonomy and evoking internal resources.
- **Power distance**: A cultural dimension from Hofstede's theory that refers to the extent to which people in a society accept and expect unequal distribution of power in relationships.
- **Self-affirmation theory**: A psychological theory suggesting that affirming core personal values can reduce defensiveness and support openness to behavior change.
- **Structural determinants of health**: Systemic and societal factors such as racism, housing, education, and access to resources that shape health outcomes and disparities.

Why Culture Matters

Imagine a nurse meeting with a patient who has been recently diagnosed with diabetes. The patient is a middle-aged Indigenous woman, who responds politely but also seems guarded and offers short responses. The nurse, trained in preventative healthcare and eager to help, begins discussing the importance of medication adherence and dietary changes that include giving up many of her favorite traditional food dishes. The nurse thinks that this visit has gone well. However, the patient doesn't return for her follow-up appointment. What do you think could have gone wrong here? The clinic's social worker reaches out and learns that the patient did not return for follow-up because the patient had deep concerns rooted in her cultural beliefs, distrust of the healthcare system, and a desire to consult her tribal elders before making decisions about treatment. What was missing in the encounter wasn't clinical knowledge or care and a desire to help on the part of the nurse; it was cultural attunement and developing trust with the patient.

In healthcare, we will find that unless our interactions with patients are delivered in a way that respects each patient's individuality, identity, and values they will fall flat. **Culture** is at the heart of who we are and shapes how we understand health and illness, how we seek help, and how we make decisions (Rice & Liamputtong, 2023). **Motivational interviewing** already emphasizes partnership, compassion, **evocation**, and empowerment, offering a powerful framework for bridging cultural gaps in clinical care. As we will see throughout this chapter, this work requires more than learning about "other" cultures; it demands reflection on our own social positioning, biases, and assumptions. It asks us to shift from being experts who fix to being listeners who partner, from a place of cultural understanding and a willingness to allow the patient to tell us who they are, how they see the world, and what changes, if any, that they would like to embark upon *with* you related to their health.

Historical Context: Exploitation and Segregation in U.S. Healthcare

For much of modern history, Western healthcare systems have been rooted in Eurocentric, biomedical models of care (Paton et al., 2020). These models often ignored and devalued cultural beliefs, traditional healing practices, and community knowledge related to health and healing. This exclusion cannot be written off as a mere oversight; rather, it was frequently coupled with systemic discrimination, exploitation, and abuse of marginalized populations.

In the United States, numerous examples illustrate how racial and ethnic minorities have been harmed in the name of science and public health throughout the history of healthcare in our country. These include the Tuskegee syphilis study, when black males were deceived and denied treatment (Gamble, 1997); the forced sterilizations of Indigenous, Black, and Latina women without their consent (Patel, 2017); the use of Henrietta Lack's cervical cancer cells without consent (Baptiste et al., 2022), and the more wide-spread exploitation of immigrant and low-income communities for clinical trials or inadequate care (Elliott & Abadie, 2008; Hacker et al., 2015; Ortega et al., 2007). These violations were often justified under the guise of medical advancement or population control, and they have left lasting legacies of mistrust that persist within these populations today.

In addition to these experiences, the roots of health care inequities in the United States are deeply intwined with the country's history of racial segregation, discriminatory policies, and systemic oppression. During the Jim Crow era, segregation laws explicitly denied Black Americans access to equal health care facilities, medical education, and services (Williams & Jackson, 2005). Black patients were routinely relegated to separate, often substandard hospital wings or denied treatment altogether. In many regions, where hospitals refused to admit Black patients, individuals had to rely on underfunded and overcrowded facilities and to develop and utilize more informal community-based forms of treatment.

Even after the formal end of legal segregation, with implementation of the Civil Rights Act of 1964, racial disparities persisted through institutional racism, biased clinical decision-making, and unequal access to insurance and preventive care. Similar patterns of exclusion and mistreatment affected Native American, Latine, and Asian American communities, as well as people with disabilities, immigrants, and members of the LGBTQIA+ population.

This storied history of discrimination has resulted in long-standing **health disparities**:

- Higher rates of infant and maternal mortality among Black and Indigenous populations (Jang & Lee, 2022)
- Disproportionate burdens of chronic illnesses, such as diabetes and hypertension (Ogunniyi et al., 2021; Yedjou et al., 2024)
- Unequal treatment for pain, mental health conditions, and substance use disorders (Hirani et al., 2024; McGuire & Miranda, 2008; Vargas et al., 2025; Wright, 2025)
- Lower life expectancy and access to specialty care in racially minoritized communities (Hill & Artiga, 2023; Nass et al., 2024).

These disparities are not exclusively the result of individual bias in healthcare, but they are reflective of **structural determinants of health** in society that have been present throughout history in the United States, such as housing, education, environmental exposures, epigenetics, and access to nutritious food. All these factors have been shaped by historic and ongoing policies rooted in racism and exclusion.

Understanding this history is crucial for providers who use MI with all patients, especially those who are from marginalized communities. Without recognizing how structural barriers, **medical mistrust**, and **historical trauma** shape patient's beliefs, behaviors, and trust surrounding health care interactions, the application of MI may be applied in a culturally tone-deaf, ineffective manner.

Culturally responsive MI goes beyond surface-level adjustments. It acknowledges that for many patients, especially those from historically excluded groups, healthcare is not just about personal motivation; it is about navigating systems that were never built to serve them. Therefore, providers must approach MI with deep awareness of power dynamics, historical harm, and the resilience and strength of communities that have long advocated for their own health and well-being, often in the face of adversity.

Defining Culture: From Cultural Competency to Cultural Humility

What do we mean when we talk about *culture* in a health care setting? Culture is more than a person's ethnicity, language, or religious affiliation. Culture is the deeply rooted system of beliefs, values, practices, and worldviews that shape how people experience and find meaning in their lives. This includes their health. What bigger part of life do we have than our health? Health is interpreted differently for different people and within different cultures, just as suffering and healing hold different meanings for different people and within different cultures. Culture influences everything from how a patient interprets their symptoms to who they trust for advice and how they define "getting better."

Culture is not just one thing. Rather it is dynamic and multifaceted. Culture is influenced by race, ethnicity, gender identity, sexual orientation, nationality, immigration history, education, religion, language, disability status, and socioeconomic status. Additionally, many people hold more than one intersecting identity, and all these identities come together to make them unique. This is known as the concept of **intersectionality**. Individuals cannot be reduced to one, single demographic or cultural label. Examples of intersectionality include the following:

- A Black, transgender woman navigating HIV care: She may face racism in medical systems, transphobia from providers, and stigma related to HIV. Her intersecting identities may increase medical mistrust and reduce the likelihood of engaging in preventative care. Being aware of all these layers when working with this patient would help to build rapport, understanding, and support the patient in making decisions related to health care.
- An undocumented Latina single mother living with diabetes: She may experience fear of deportation, limited access to insurance, language barriers, and cultural expectations around family and food. Her experiences of marginalization are shaped by the intersection of immigration status, socioeconomic class, gender, and ethnicity. A provider might focus on family-centered motivations and explore culturally meaningful approaches to health while also affirming her resilience and resourcefulness.
- An elderly White male living in a rural area with PTSD: While this patient may benefit from some social privilege as a White male, he is also living in a location that can be isolating and may limit his access to resources. Additionally, his mental health status may create barriers to care. His identity as a veteran may also influence his views on autonomy, strength, and help seeking. A provider could affirm his self-reliance while exploring how accepting support aligns with values like protecting his family or being strong for others.

Another factor to consider is that two patients who both belong to the same cultural group may have differing identities and views. For example, two patients that both identify as Latine might have very different relationships to language, family, trauma, or spirituality that are based on their personal histories and social contexts. Think about others in your own life who have cultural similarities to you and ask yourself if you see things in the exact same way as those individuals or if there are differences.

Over the past several decades, health care institutions have recognized that cultural misunderstandings and biases contribute to disparities in treatment and outcomes. This gave rise to the concept of **cultural competency**, an effort to prepare providers with knowledge about different cultural groups to improve communication and care. While this was a step forward, it often took a static, checklist approach, encouraging providers to learn about other cultures as if they were all the same and belonged to fixed or predictable categories. "If I have an Asian patient, I can expect this and should act in this way. If I have a Black patient, they will be like this, and I should do this." This had the inadvertent effect of reinforcing stereotypes and overlooking the uniqueness of each patient's lived experience.

In response to the cultural competency model, many have shifted toward a model of **cultural humility**. A term coined by Drs. Melanie Tervalon and Jann Murray-García (1998), "cultural humility" is not an endpoint but a lifelong process of self-reflection and a commitment to understanding the power imbalances in the patient-provider relationship. Rather than aiming for mastery or competency over another person's culture, cultural humility encourages providers to do the following:

- Recognize and reflect on one's own cultural identity and biases
- Approach each patient with curiosity and openness
- Acknowledge systemic inequities and how they impact health
- Share power in the clinical encounter

Motivational interviewing inherently supports the concept of cultural humility (Lee, 2025). It asks clinicians to suspend judgment, to listen deeply, and to affirm the patient's autonomy and expertise in their own life, and finally to empower patients to make decisions for themselves. Practicing MI through a lens of cultural humility means being tuned in, not only to what the patient is telling you but also to what their words mean within their cultural framework. It also means being willing to acknowledge when we, as providers, might not have the same background and understanding as our patients and that we must also be open to learning *from* our patients about who they are.

An example of this might include a nurse who is working with a 70-year-old Black male who has recently hospitalized for heart failure and is now being encouraged to reduce sodium intake and take several daily medications. The nurse notices that the patient seems polite but disengaged, and during their conversation he states, "I've lived through a lot worse than this, and I've gotten by without all of these pills so far." Rather than immediately assuming that the patient is resistant, a culturally humble approach would involve listening for the deeper context. Through use of open-ended questions and reflective statements the provider learns that the patient has lived through the civil rights era, experienced medical racism firsthand, and both he and his family have a long-standing mistrust in the healthcare system. Instead of correcting or persuading, the provider reflects: "You've had to rely on your own strength and judgment for a long time, especially in systems that have not always treated you fairly. It makes sense that you'd feel cautious about putting trust in medication right now. Would it be okay if we talked about what concerns you most and what matters most to you going forward?" This response does several important things:

- It acknowledges the historical and personal context that the patient has experienced and how that influences the patient's worldview.
- It expresses respect for autonomy and resilience rather than challenges it.
- It invites collaboration, creating a space for shared decision-making grounded in mutual respect.

By honoring cultural identity and lived experiences, MI becomes more than a behavior change strategy; it becomes a means of restoring agency, dignity, and trust into a system that has often failed to provide it for those who need it most.

Cultural Influences on Health Behavior and Communication

Health decisions do not occur in a vacuum. They are shaped by the cultural values, norms, and communication styles that influence how people understand illness, relate to providers, and make choices about care. For practitioners using MI, recognizing these cultural influences is essential to building rapport, eliciting meaningful **change talk**, and ensuring the process is respectful and effective. Let's explore several key cultural dimensions that commonly influence health behavior and patient-provider interactions.

Family Roles, Community Decision-Making, and Health Beliefs

In many cultures, health decisions are not made by individuals alone, but in consultation with family members, elders, or trusted community leaders. Remember, it is important not to stereotype all individuals from one culture as holding the same beliefs, but you may find the following:

- In many Indigenous communities, decisions are made collectively, with deep respect for tribal traditions and elder wisdom.

- In Latine, Asian, and Middle Eastern cultures, family members may be closely involved in decisions around treatment, disclosure, or end-of-life care.
- In Black communities, the church or extended kin networks may play an influential role in shaping health behaviors and norms.

When working with patients, it is important to explore who the patient sees as key influences in their life. Rather than making assumptions, providers can ask these questions:

- Who do you usually talk to when you're making decisions about your health?
- Are there family or community members you'd like to include in this conversation?

Acknowledging these dynamics shows cultural humility, a willingness to let the patient lead, and invites partnership between patient and provider.

The Role of Spirituality in Shaping Beliefs About Health

Spirituality is a central guiding force in many people's understandings of health and illness. Patients may view illness as a test of faith, a punishment or spiritual imbalance, or a sacred opportunity for growth and transformation. For example, you may encounter some patients who say things like "If it's God's will, I will be healed." We may interpret this as passive, but when we look at it through a cultural lens, statements like these may reflect a deep spiritual trust and surrender instead of a lack of motivation.

In connection with this, fatalism, or the belief that events are predetermined and out of one's control, can influence health behaviors, particularly in communities that have experienced historical trauma or chronic marginalization. Rather than trying to "correct" these beliefs, MI invites providers to partner with and explore them. Some good questions to ask are these:

- How do your spiritual beliefs guide the choices you make about your health?
- What do you feel that you can control in this situation? What do you feel is out of your control?

Another factor that varies within cultures is time orientation. Some cultures prioritize living for the present moment and view future planning as less important. This could impact readiness to engage in long-term plans or preventive care. Rather than viewing this as a lack of motivation for change, seek to learn about it from a place of gaining a better understanding of your patient's worldview. Exploring values and linking behavior change to immediate or relational benefits like being present for grandchildren or staying active to continue engaging in important roles they may have in the community may be more effective than trying to convince patients of the importance of planning for long-term outcomes.

Power Distance and Patient Autonomy

Power distance is a concept that originates from the work of Geert Hofstede's (1980) cultural dimensions theory, and it refers to how cultures tolerate unequal distributions of power in relationships, like those found between teacher and student or patient and provider. In high-power distance cultures (many Asian, Middle Eastern, and Latin American cultures) patients may expect that the provider be directive and authoritative. Questioning or disagreeing with the one in power may be seen as disrespectful. In low-power distance cultures (the United States, Australia, Europe), patients are more likely to view the patient-provider relationship as collaborative. Patients may expect to be more involved in decision-making and to share an open dialogue.

MI, which emphasizes patient autonomy, collaboration, and partnership, may need to be adapted when working with patients from high-power distance cultures to build trust and credibility. Providers can still use MI principles like empathy, evoking patient values, and affirming personal agency, but providers may need to hold more formal tones and to respect the hierarchical framework that the patient is comfortable with. This might look like this: "I have some recommendations, but what's most important is how they fit with your life and beliefs. Would it be helpful to talk through that together?" If the patient seems resistant to engage, it is okay for the provider to offer their recommendations from a more traditional expert approach.

High-Context versus Low-Context Communication Styles

Another cultural factor that influences health care communication is the distinction between **high-context communication** and **low-context communication**. These are concepts that were first introduced by Edward T. Hall (1976), who is a founding figure in intercultural communication theory. These concepts have been applied widely in health care, counseling, business, and education settings to understand how people from various cultures convey meaning. High-context cultures value indirect communication, nonverbal cues, shared social knowledge, and subtlety. Low-context cultures prioritize directness, explicitness, and clarity in speech.

Table 10.1 Communication styles

High-Context Communication	Low-Context Communication
Indirect, implicit	Direct, explicit

High-Context Communication	Low-Context Communication
Relies on nonverbal cues	Relies on verbal expression
Meaning tied to context and relationships	Meaning tied to words themselves
Common in collectivist cultures	Common in individualist cultures
Examples: Japan, Arab countries, and many Indigenous countries	Examples: United States, Germany, Scandinavia

Patients from high-context cultures may avoid direct disagreement, downplay their distress, or use indirect language to express ambivalence. In MI, this requires attentive listening on the part of the provider, comfort with silence, and sensitivity to tone and body language. Open-ended questions like the following allow for gentle exploration without demanding confrontation:

- What's your sense of how things are going?
- What do you wish your provider understood better about your experience?

In contrast, patients from low-context cultures may value direct, clear, and efficient conversations. MI can remain rational while being more linear and goal oriented in these contexts. Understanding communication styles is another way to allow patients to educate us on who they are and understand their world view. Approaching patients in a way that is respectful of their preferred communication style can help providers to create a more authentic space for conversations. This not only builds trust but also increases the likelihood that behavior change plans will be meaningful, respectful, and sustainable.

Culturally Adapted Motivational Interviewing and Beyond

Defining culture can seem both simple and complex. Often when we think of the word "culture" we may think of someone's traditions, the holidays they celebrate, or the foods that they eat (Lee, 2025). This is part of what makes up someone's culture, but there is a lot more to it than that. Dr. Christina S. Lee of the Boston University School of Social Work developed **culturally adapted motivational interviewing (CAMI)**, and she offers the following definition of culture: "Culture is … *what matters* to a person, their everyday priorities" (Lee, 2025, p. 13). We often fall into stereotypes when it comes to culture and assume that because someone belongs to one cultural group that they must embody certain qualities that we have heard or seen amongst others of that group, but true cultural awareness understands that culture is personal. What culture means to one person is not the same as what it means to someone else, and culture is evolving. It is not stagnant. For example, the concept of machismo, or a strong sense of masculine pride, can be found in some Latin cultures, but that does not mean that all people within that cultural group espouse the values of machismo. There are differences from person to person and from generation to generation. As society changes so do people.

Lee (2025) emphasizes adapting MI to work effectively across diverse cultural contexts. She teaches that while the spirit of MI, partnership, acceptance, compassion, and evocation, is universally applicable, practitioners must also remain flexible and culturally responsive in order to meet their patients where they are. Some of the key techniques and strategies outlined in CAMI are as follows:

- Affirming cultural identity: Embedding **cultural strengths** and values into reflections and affirmations so that clients feel their background is a resource, not a barrier, to change.
- Strengthening rapport: Building trust by demonstrating a genuine curiosity about a person's cultural worldview, using open-ended questions, reflections, and culturally tailored language and idioms.
- Asking about culture without stereotyping: Inviting clients to describe what their culture means to them rather than relying on assumptions, through neutral, respectful probes (e.g., "What cultural practices give you strength?)
- Exploring experiences of stigma and discrimination: Gently eliciting change talk by inviting discussion of past or ongoing bias (e.g., "How has 'x' affected your health goals?"), then linking those experiences to motivation for change.
- Linking social/structural determinants: Highlighting connections between broader factors (e.g., access to care, economic stressors, systemic racism) and personal health behaviors to deepen discrepancy and evoke commitment.
- Sociocultural stressors and disparities: Recognizing and naming specific community-level stressors (e.g., immigration stress, intergenerational trauma) as legitimate parts of the conversation, thereby validating the client experience and fostering collaboration).
- Reflecting on your own cultural biases: It is important for clinicians to reflect on and check their own cultural assumptions before proceeding.

CAMI can be used as a culturally responsive decision-making tool by embedding cultural awareness at every step. From engagement to goal setting to sustaining change, it enables more ethical, effective, and inclusive care, especially when working across differences in race, ethnicity, language, and belief systems. Lee (2025) talks about the skill of evocation being referred to as "the heart of MI." With traditional MI we work to evoke the patient's own motivations and reasons for change and to draw out this motivation by getting the patient to engage in change talk, using their own words to move them forward toward change. Lee (2025) says that the "heart of CAMI" is "evocation for empowerment" (p. 25). We focus on empowerment as a way to affirm and support the individual in their own journey toward change. Lee feels that we can view CAMI as traditional MI in combination with **self-affirmation theory**.

MI evolved out of humanistic counseling, so instead of viewing others as operating from a place of deficit, being broken, or in need of fixing, those who apply MI look at people as rich with internal resources that merely need to be tapped into and drawn out. Practitioners adopting an MI stance seek to evoke motivation and wisdom from within the client rather than impose change externally onto the client. The approach is strengths based, collaborative, and focused on honoring the individual's own values, goals, and decision-making process.

CAMI builds on this foundation by explicitly integrating cultural identity, lived experience, and systemic context into the patient-provider conversation. CAMI not only avoids pathologizing culturally rooted behaviors or beliefs, but it actively seeks to leverage cultural strengths such as family support systems, spiritual traditions, and collective resilience as powerful sources of motivation and healing. Rather than treating culture as a barrier to engagement or behavior change, CAMI reframes it as a tool for connection, insight, and empowerment. This approach recognizes that meaningful and sustainable change is most likely to occur when it aligns with the client's cultural worldview, values, and community ties. In both traditional MI and CAMI, the practitioner's role is not to "fix" the client but to foster a safe, respectful space where change talk can emerge, guided by curiosity, compassion, and cultural humility.

Reflecting on Bias and Power in Motivational Interviewing

To practice MI with cultural responsiveness, practitioners must begin with self-reflection. This involves intentionally examining how one's own cultural background, social identities, and life experiences shape perceptions of others and influence clinical interactions. Start by considering the visible and invisible aspects of your identity, things like race, ethnicity, gender, sexual orientation, socioeconomic status, age, religion, ability, and language. Reflect on which of these identities feel most central to your daily experience. Then, ask yourself, "In what contexts do I experience privilege? Where might I face marginalization? How might these dynamics affect the way I relate to clients whose identities differ from my own? How might the client feel based upon their cultural identity versus mine?"

Next, consider how these identities and experiences might influence your communication style, assumptions about change, and perceptions of client resistance or readiness. Reflecting on implicit biases can help uncover patterns that may inadvertently shape clinical judgments. We all have **implicit bias**, whether we are aware of it or not. Implicit biases are the unconscious beliefs that we carry about others. Ask yourself what stereotypes you might have internalized about certain groups? How might these show up in your tone, body language, or word choice when using MI with patients?

Harvard University offers an implicit association test (IAT), which will help you assess internal biases related to race, gender, and age. You can take the test through Harvard's Project Implicit at implicit.harvard.edu/implicit/takeatest.html. You can also assess your automatic reactions and internal biases related to mental health and substance use disorders by going to projectimplicithealth.com/. These are great places to start that can give you an idea of your internal biases so that you can reflect and work to address them within your patient interactions.

Research on MI and Cultural Considerations

While there is still room for research on MI and various cultural and minority groups, we do have some to support the effectiveness of applying MI cross culturally. MI was originally developed in North America and Europe but has since been taught and utilized in many different languages and nations throughout the world. Miller and Rollnick (2023) state that in the United States MI outcomes have been at least as good or better for minority groups as compared to White-majority populations, citing that it is well suited to working with culturally diverse populations with its high emphasis on empathy and acceptance and with clients being viewed with cultural humility as MI teaches practitioners to view clients as the experts on themselves.

A systematic review of 25 peer-reviewed CAMI studies over 20 years was conducted by Self et al. (2022) showed that 10 out of 17 RCTs with control groups reported CAMI outperforming standard MI on primary outcomes. These adaptations typically involved customizing "context, content, and concepts" to align with participants cultural values, three of the dimensions of cultural adaptation defined by the **ecological validity framework** developed by Bernal et al. in 1995. ***Context*** refers to the setting, social environment, and delivery mechanisms of the MI intervention, which includes where and how MI is delivered (e.g., community centers, clinics, churches, homes), the language used and the demographics of the practitioner (e.g., cultural or racial matching), and historical or sociopolitical factors relevant to the population (e.g., colonialism, mistrust of institutions, and immigration experiences). The goal with context is to create a culturally safe and relevant environment for the intervention to be received. ***Content*** refers to the specific messages, metaphors, and examples used in the MI sessions. This includes topics discussed and how they are framed (e.g., referencing family obligations versus individual autonomy), values-based language (e.g., honoring ancestors, being a good role model, or respecting elders), and narratives or analogies that are culturally familiar (e.g., storytelling and spiritual idioms). The goal with content is to ensure the material resonates with the client's lived experience and value system. ***Concepts*** refer to the underlying cultural beliefs, values, and explanatory models related to health, behavior, and change. This includes ideas about illness, addiction, healing, and responsibility along with spiritual or religious beliefs that influence motivation and decision-making and cultural views of family roles, interdependence, fatalism, or collectivism versus individualism. The goal with concepts is to align the motivational strategies of MI with the population's worldview and cognitive frameworks for understanding behavior.

While Millner and Rollnick (2023) and Lee (2025) support the use of MI effectively among various minority groups and cultures, research is still emerging. Much of the current research consists mostly of secondary data analyses, pilot trials, and mixed-methods studies. More large-scale, controlled, and comparative research is needed to fully establish MI's effectiveness across intersectional identities. As with all scientific inquiry, it is important to recognize that we do not prove theories definitively; rather, we accumulate evidence that supports or challenges them. In the case of MI, while current research offers encouraging findings when it comes to cultural applications, we cannot assert its effectiveness with certainty across all contexts. Thus, caution is warranted when generalizing outcomes. Nonetheless, the relational foundations and adaptability of MI do provide a promising framework for culturally responsive practice, especially when implemented with careful attention to context, identity, and lived experience.

Where to Go From Here: Cultural Responsiveness in Real Time

Applying MI in high-demand health care environments such as hospitals, emergency departments, and outpatient clinics may initially appear impractical due to time constraints, documentation deadlines and requirements, and the urgency of medical decision-making. However, MI, does not need to be a lengthy intervention in order to have an impact. When used with intentionality and cultural awareness, even brief moments of MI can enhance patient engagement, build trust, and increase collaboration between provider and patient across diverse populations.

Research supports the efficacy of brief MI interventions, sometimes lasting as little as 5–15 minutes, particularly in areas such as medication adherence, chronic disease management, smoking cessation, and behavior change. When patients feel that their provider is respectful, empathic, and attuned to their cultural values, they will be more likely to disclose concerns, express ambivalence, and participate actively in treatment planning. In multicultural hospital settings, where mistrust and miscommunication may be heightened and mostly likely to occur, a culturally responsive MI approach can bridge gaps in understanding and restore a sense of agency for the patient.

Practical Strategies for Busy Providers

1. Use the spirit of MI, not just the techniques. MI is not only a set of tools but a way of being. In time-limited interactions, leading with partnership, acceptance, compassion, and evocation can shift the tone of even brief conversations. A warm greeting, validation of the patient's concerns, or respectful acknowledgment of cultural or linguistic differences can create an opening for collaboration.

   Example: "I know you may have had challenging healthcare experiences in the past, but I want to make sure I understand what matters most to you right now."

2. Affirm cultural values and strengths. When patients express hesitation, resistance, or uncertainty, MI invites providers to explore the deeper values behind those concerns. For culturally diverse populations, affirming collectivist values, spiritual frameworks, or intergenerational decision-making norms can deepen rapport and reframe change as aligned with, not in opposition to, their individual culture and identity.

   Example: "It sounds like your family plays a big role in your health decisions. How have they helped you through difficult times in the past?"

3. Evoke, don't prescribe. In high-pressure clinical settings it can be tempting to default to telling patients what to do. Instead, use open-ended questions and reflections to elicit the patient's own reasoning and motivation. When patients are heard, especially those from marginalized backgrounds who may feel overlooked, judged, or like they have not had a voice in the past, they are more likely to engage meaningfully. This can be a huge step toward building trust.

   Example: Provider offers a quick MI Prompt: "What concerns you most about your current condition?" Follow-up: "What would help you feel more in control right now?"

4. Reflect and reframe from a cultural lens. Skillful reflections can acknowledge not just what the person is saying, but also their cultural and emotional frame. Reframing resistance as cultural wisdom or survival can reduce shame, increase openness to dialogue, and foster understanding and connection between provider and patient.

   Example: "It makes sense that you'd be cautions because you've seen others in your community struggle with this too. It sounds like you want to protect yourself and your family."

KEY POINTS

- Culture is not separate from MI. It is intricately woven into how MI is practiced and understood.
- MI stems from humanistic counseling, emphasizing autonomy, empathy, and seeing the client as the expert on their own life, all principles that align well with culturally informed care.
- The field is shifting from cultural competency (a static checklist) to cultural humility, a lifelong, reflective process of learning, openness, and power sharing.
- Intersectionality shapes patient experience. Patients hold multiple identities that influence their health care experiences, and providers must consider how these intersect to create unique challenges and strengths.
- Historical trauma and structural inequities matter. Medical mistrust, discrimination, and systemic oppression have long impacted marginalized communities, and these realities must be acknowledged in clinical care.
- Cultural beliefs influence health behavior and decision-making. Family roles, spirituality, time orientation, and communication style are all culturally influenced and should be respected and explored in MI.
- Power distance and communication styles vary across cultures. Some patients expect directive providers; others expect collaboration. MI must be adapted accordingly, without losing its core spirit.
- CAMI offers a framework for cultural adaptation and helps providers affirm identity, explore sociocultural stressors, and tailor content to match patient worldviews and values.
- Brief MI can be powerful in clinical settings. Even in time-limited environments, short MI-informed conversations, when culturally attuned, can increase trust and patient engagement.
- Self-awareness and bias reflection are essential. Providers must engage in ongoing self-reflection about their own social positioning and internal biases to practice MI ethically and effectively.
- MI works best when patients feel heard, respected, and empowered. Empowerment, not persuasion, is the goal. MI and CAMI emphasize listening, evoking, and partnering with patients, especially those from marginalized backgrounds.
- Cultural strengths are powerful motivators for change. Drawing from cultural values, family ties, and spiritual beliefs can enhance patient motivation and help create more resonant and effective change plans.

QUESTIONS FOR REFLECTION

- How does your own cultural background and life experience influence the way you interact with patients, and how might this impact your use of MI in diverse clinical situations?
- In what ways can cultural humility differ from cultural competency in your practice, and how could adopting an attitude of humility enhance your effectiveness as a provider?
- Reflect on a time when cultural beliefs or values may have affected a patient's health decisions or engagement. How could a culturally responsive MI approach have changed the outcome?

SUGGESTED ACTIVITIES

1. Cultural identity reflection wheel. Help students examine how their cultural background and clinical roles intersect. Create a cultural identity reflection wheel including race, ethnicity, gender, language, socioeconomic background, religious or spiritual beliefs, and nursing values. Then, write a one- to two-page reflection:

    - How do my identities shape the way I communicate with patients?
    - Where might I unconsciously bring bias into clinical interactions?
    - How does my role as a nurse impact the power dynamic in patient care?

    After everyone has completed the activity, have a whole-class or small group discussion about this activity and what you have learned.
2. Cultural mistrust in health care simulation and discussion. Build empathy and awareness of structural barriers.

    - Facilitate a simulation or video case in which a patient from a historically marginalized group expresses mistrust in the healthcare system.
    - Students work in groups to create a response plan using MI principles and culturally responsive strategies.
    - Follow with a facilitated debrief on what helped or hindered trust and how a nurse's tone, presence, and questions can impact clinical outcomes.
    - *Optional:* Include short readings on the Tuskegee study or Henrietta Lacks for historical context.
3. Communication styles and cultural context. Apply high- versus low-context communication principles in nursing assessments.

- Present two patient profiles from different cultural backgrounds (e.g., a Somali elder with diabetes and a White U.S. veteran with PTSD).
- In small groups, students create two nursing communication plans, adjusting tone, phrasing, and structure based on the patient's communication style.
- Present plans to the class:
    - How did your team modify standard nursing communication to meet the needs of your patient?
    - How can cultural understanding reduce miscommunication or nonadherence?

4. CAMI application in nursing care plan. Integrate CAMI into a nursing process framework.
    - Students select a culturally diverse patient population (e.g., undocumented Latina woman, Indigenous elders, LGBTQ+ youth).
    - Using the nursing process (ADPIE: assessment, diagnosis, planning, implementation, evaluation), build a care plan that incorporates CAMI strategies:
        - Include at least one culturally adapted MI question.
        - Identify cultural strengths and barriers.
        - Propose culturally attuned nursing interventions.

    Students will either write a short care plan or give a short presentation sharing all elements.

5. Bias assessment and journal reflections. Increase student self-awareness of biases and their impact on care.
    - Students complete Harvard's Project implicit bias test online (implicit.harvard.edu/implicit/takeatest.html).
    - Answer the following journal prompt questions:
        - What did I learn about myself?
        - How might these unconscious beliefs show up in patient care?
        - How can I intentionally practice cultural humility in my nursing role?
    - *Optional:* Create a personal growth goal related to culturally responsive nursing practice.

References

Baptiste, D., Caviness-Ashe, N., Josiah, N., Commodore-Mensah, Y., Arscott, J., Wilson, P. R., & Starks, S. (2022). Henrietta lacks and America's dark history of research involving African Americans. *Nursing Open*, *9*(5), 2236–2238. https://doi.org/10.1002/nop2.1257

Bernal, G., Bonilla, J., & Bellido, C. (1995). Ecological validity and cultural sensitivity for outcome research: Issues for the cultural adaptation and development of psychosocial treatments with hispanics. *Journal of Abnormal Child Psychology, 23*(1), 67–82. https://doi.org/10.1007/bf01447045

Cain, D. J. (2010). *Humanistic psychotherapies: Handbook of research and practice*. American Psychological Association.

Elliott, C., & Abadie, R. (2008). Exploiting a research underclass in phase 1 clinical trials. *New England Journal of Medicine, 358*(22), 2316–2317. https://doi.org/10.1056/nejmp0801872

Gamble, V. N. (1997). Under the shadow of Tuskegee: African Americans and health care. *American Journal of Public Health, 87*(11), 1773–1778. https://doi.org/10.2105/ajph.87.11.1773

Hacker, K., Anies, M., Folb, B., & Zallman, L. (2015). Barriers to health care for undocumented immigrants: A literature review. *Risk Management and Healthcare Policy, 175*. https://doi.org/10.2147/rmhp.s70173

Hall, E. T. (1976). *Beyond culture*. Anchor Books.

Hill, L., & Artiga, S. (2023, May 23). *What is driving widening racial disparities in life expectancy?* Kaiser Family Foundation. https://www.kff.org/racial-equity-and-health-policy/issue-brief/what-is-driving-widening-racial-disparities-in-life-expectancy/

Hirani, S., Benkli, B., Odonkor, C., Hirani, Z., Oso, T., Bohacek, S., Wiedrick, J., Hildebrand, A., Osuagwu, U., Orhurhu, V., Hooten, W., Abdi, S., & Meghani, S. (2024). Racial disparities in opioid prescribing in the United States from 2011 to 2021: A systematic review and meta-analysis. *Journal of Pain Research, 17*, 3639–3649. https://doi.org/10.2147/jpr.s477128

Hofstede, G. (1980). *Culture's consequences: International differences in work-related values*. SAGE.

Jang, C., & Lee, H. (2022). A review of racial disparities in infant mortality in the us. *Children, 9*(2), 257. https://doi.org/10.3390/children9020257

Lee, C. S. (2025). *Motivational interviewing across cultures: Optimizing practice*. Guilford Press.

McGuire, T. G., & Miranda, J. (2008). New evidence regarding racial and ethnic disparities in mental health: Policy implications. *Health Affairs, 27*(2), 393–403. https://doi.org/10.1377/hlthaff.27.2.393

Miller, W. R., & Rollnick, S. (2013). *Motivational interviewing: Helping people change* (3rd ed.). Guilford Press.

Miller, W. R., & Rollnick, S. (2023). *Motivational interviewing: Helping people change and grow* (4th ed.). Guilford Press.

Nass, S. J., Amankwah, F. K., & DeVoe, J. E. (Eds.). (2024). *Ending unequal treatment: Strategies to achieve equitable health care and optimal health for all*. National Academies Press. https://www.ncbi.nlm.nih.gov/books/NBK607572/

North, A., & Alarik, S. (2022). *Person-centered therapy (Rogerian therapy)*. StatPearls. https://www.ncbi.nlm.nih.gov/books/NBK589708/

Ogunniyi, M. O., Commodore-Mensah, Y., & Ferdinand, K. C. (2021). Race, ethnicity, hypertension, and heart disease. *Journal of the American College of Cardiology, 78*(24), 2460–2470. https://doi.org/10.1016/j.jacc.2021.06.017

Ortega, A. N., Fang, H., Perez, V. H., Rizzo, J. A., Carter-Pokras, O., Wallace, S. P., & Gelberg, L. (2007). Health care access, use of services, and experiences among undocumented Mexicans and other Latinos. *Archives of Internal Medicine, 167*(21), 2354. https://doi.org/10.1001/archinte.167.21.2354

Patel, P. (2017). Forced sterilization of women as discrimination. *Public Health Reviews, 38*(1). https://doi.org/10.1186/s40985-017-0060-9

Paton, M., Naidu, T., Wyatt, T. R., Oni, O., Lorello, G. R., Najeeb, U., Feilchenfeld, Z., Waterman, S. J., Whitehead, C., & Kuper, A. (2020). Dismantling the master's house: New ways of knowing for equity and social justice in health professions education. *Advances in Health Sciences Education, 25*(5). https://doi.org/10.1007/s10459-020-10006-x

Rice, Z. S., & Liamputtong, P. (2023). Cultural determinants of health, cross-cultural research and global public health. In P. Liamputtong (Ed.), *Handbook of social sciences and global public health* (pp. 1–14). Springer. https://doi.org/10.1007/978-3-030-96778-9_44-1

Rogers, C. R. (1951). *Client-centered therapy: Its current practice, implications and theory.* Houghton Mifflin.

Rogers, C. R. (1961). *On becoming a person: A therapist's view of psychotherapy.* Houghton Mifflin.

Self, K. J., Borsari, B., Ladd, B. O., Nicolas, G., Gibson, C. J., Jackson, K., & Manuel, J. K. (2023). Cultural adaptations of motivational interviewing: A systematic review. *Psychological Services, 20*(Suppl 1), 7–18. https://doi.org/10.1037/ser0000619

Tervalon, M., & Murray-García, J. (1998). Cultural humility versus cultural competence: A critical distinction in defining physician training outcomes in multicultural education. *Journal of Health Care for the Poor and Underserved, 9*(2), 117–125. https://doi.org/10.1353/hpu.2010.0233

Vargas, A., Tobey-Moore, L., Curran, G., Elkhateb, R., Sexton, K., Bailey, B., Nagel, C., & Goree, J. (2025). Exploring racial disparities in chronic pain management. *Journal of Pain Research, 18*, 2901–2908. https://doi.org/10.2147/jpr.s493664

Williams, D. R., & Jackson, P. B. (2005). Social sources of racial disparities in health. *Health Affairs, 24*(2), 325–334.

Wright, M. F. (2025). Racial disparities in outpatient substance use disorder treatment completion: Trends and changes from 2004 to 2024. *International Journal of Environmental Research and Public Health, 22*(2), 278. https://doi.org/10.3390/ijerph22020278

Yedjou, C. G., Sims, J. N., NJiki, S., Chitoh, A. M., Joseph, M., Cherkos, A. S., & Tchounwou, P. B. (2024). Health and racial disparities in diabetes mellitus prevalence, management, policies, and outcomes in the United States. *Journal of Community Medicine & Public Health, 8*(3). https://doi.org/10.29011/2577-2228.100460

Epilogue

Motivational interviewing is an evidence-based counseling technique that has been shown to help patients make lifestyle changes. It puts ownership of health back into the hands of the patient, where it should be. It empowers patients to take charge of their health. It moves us from being patient centered to allowing patients to drive their own health without fear of judgment from us. For the provider it is a liberating experience. Society and insurance entities make us feel like we are responsible for curing our patients, but the reality is much of what will cure them lies within their control, not ours. Providers suffer from burnout by not being able to meet these unrealistic expectations, feeling as if somehow, they failed their patients. We must embrace the truth that our fellow counselors have known for years that the only person who can change a patient's life is the person themselves. Helping health professionals move from a health expert to a health guide is liberating. Yes, we are the experts in the room when it comes to how the body works and what the available treatments are. Yes, we can educate our patients, but only when the patients are ready to hear it. Education alone does not change lifestyle outcomes.

As nurses and providers, we must realize that our patients have the right to make good and bad choices. They may find some habits impossible to break, and we must accept that. Unconditional positive regard accepts patients for who they are and holds them in a positive light, even if they are struggling, and even if they do not agree with our treatment plan. Unconditional positive regard never gives up on a patient. It means that we keep believing. Learning these techniques does not come easy. Research has shown that the earlier we start teaching MI skills the more time and opportunity nurses and health care providers will have to hone them. We know that providers are ambivalent to making changes in their practice, and that is okay. Research has shown that with frequent opportunities for training and ongoing support, the easier it becomes for providers to become comfortable with MI. However, this change does not happen overnight. Once providers and patients begin to see the benefits of this technique it becomes easier to implement, which takes me back to one of the very first articles I read when a provider learned MI techniques and began to implement them. She said that MI helped her to "[fall] back in love with the practice of medicine." I can relate to her sentiment. Learning MI has helped me connect with patients in a much more real and authentic way. I see patients now for who they are and what they want to be, not what I want for them. It has made me a much more effective provider, and my patients have been much more engaged. I am not going to say that I have not slipped back into the expert mode, but when I do I remind myself to respect my patients' right to choose and right to determine what type of life they want to live, including the changes they may or may not want to make in their life.

Teaching MI skills can begin with the first courses of nursing school in health promotion classes. These techniques can then be threaded throughout the remainder of student education to allow for them to develop and practice the skills. Advance practice classes can take these skills one step further to incorporate how a provider would apply them in practice, and health care organizations can provide ongoing training and support. It is a paradigm shift in healthcare to meet your patients where they are, explore with them where they want to go, and then help them get there—a much more dynamic humanistic approach that in my opinion and based on the evidence will yield a much more effective healthcare system than our present-day approach.

As you close this book and step back into your clinical practice or studies, we challenge you to be the catalyst for change in your own health care environment. Start today—commit to one conversation during which you intentionally apply the spirit and techniques of MI. Listen to your patient and let them tell their story, honor your patient's autonomy, and embrace the discomfort that comes with letting go of the expert role. Advocate for ongoing MI training in your workplace and support your colleagues as they, too, navigate this shift. Remember, lasting transformation in healthcare begins with one provider, one patient, and one authentic, collaborative conversation at a time. Will you be the one who helps your patients—and yourself—fall back in love with the healing profession? The journey starts with you.

Index